CORONARY HEART DISEASE

Gary Gerstenblith, M.D.

and

Simeon Margolis, M.D., Ph.D.

JOHNS HOPKINS MEDICINE

Dear Reader:

This is an exciting time in the field of cardiology. Last year, the U.S. Food and Drug Administration approved a new class of drugs for the treatment of heart failure and a new type of stent for preventing restenosis after angioplasty. In addition, researchers recently started investigating cell transplants for regenerating heart tissue after a heart attack, and the results so far are promising.

If you are one of the nearly 13 million Americans living with coronary heart disease, reading this White Paper will help you manage your illness; reduce your risk of complications such as heart attack, heart failure, and cardiac arrest; and improve your quality of life.

Here are some of this year's highlights:

- Yet another reason to get an annual **flu shot**. (page 11)
- Are you eating the best fish sources of **omega-3 fatty acids** for your heart? (page 32)
- A simple way to **add years to your life**. (page 35)
- Should you be taking not just one, but **two cholesterol-lowering drugs**? (page 41)
- When **aspirin** doesn't reduce your risk of a heart attack. (page 47)
- What you need to know about using **nitrate medications** to manage angina. (page 52)
- Is it safer to perform **bypass surgery on a beating heart**? (page 56)
- **Home defibrillators and wearable defibrillators** can save lives. (page 72)

I hope that by putting these advances into practice, people with, or at risk for, coronary heart disease may be able to live longer and more productive lives.

Sincerely,

Gary Gerstenblith, M.D.
Professor of Medicine
Cardiology Division, Johns Hopkins University School of Medicine

P. S. Don't forget to visit www.HopkinsAfter50.com for the latest news on coronary heart disease and other information that will complement your Johns Hopkins White Paper.

THE AUTHORS

Gary Gerstenblith, M.D., received his B.A. from New York University and his M.D. from the University of Pennsylvania School of Medicine. He performed his internship and residency at the Hospital of the University of Pennsylvania and received his cardiology training at the National Institutes of Health and the University of Miami School of Medicine. He is a professor of medicine in the division of cardiology at the Johns Hopkins University School of Medicine and is on the full-time staff at Johns Hopkins Hospital.

■ ■ ■

Simeon Margolis, M.D., Ph.D., received his M.D. and Ph.D. from the Johns Hopkins University School of Medicine and performed his internship and residency at Johns Hopkins Hospital. He is currently a professor of medicine and biological chemistry at the Johns Hopkins University School of Medicine and medical editor of *The Johns Hopkins Medical Letter: Health After 50.* He has served on various committees for the Department of Health, Education, and Welfare, including the National Diabetes Advisory Board and the Arteriosclerosis Specialized Centers of Research Review Committees. In addition, he has acted as a member of the Endocrinology and Metabolism Panel of the U.S. Food and Drug Administration.

A former weekly columnist for *The Baltimore Sun,* Dr. Margolis lectures regularly to medical students, physicians, and the general public on a wide variety of topics, such as the prevention of coronary heart disease, the control of cholesterol levels, the treatment of diabetes, and the use of alternative medicine.

CONTENTS

CORONARY HEART DISEASE

The heart is a muscular organ that pumps oxygen- and nutrient-rich blood to all the tissues of the body. To function properly, the heart also requires a supply of oxygenated blood from the coronary arteries, which encircle the top of the heart like a crown (a "corona").

In coronary heart disease (CHD), sometimes called coronary artery disease, the coronary arteries are narrowed by atherosclerosis—a buildup of deposits called plaques within the artery walls. Atherosclerosis jeopardizes the ability of the coronary arteries to provide adequate blood to the heart.

CHD is the leading cause of mortality in the United States, responsible for more than one in five deaths—nearly 700,000 a year. It can lead to several complications, including angina, heart attacks, heart failure, and arrhythmias. These last two conditions are often, but not always, a result of CHD.

Angina. Angina, also called angina pectoris, refers to episodes of chest pain due to an inadequate supply of blood to the heart. Angina affects about 6.6 million Americans.

Heart attacks. A heart attack, technically known as a myocardial infarction, refers to tissue death (infarction) due to an insufficient blood supply to portions of the heart muscle (myocardium). Approximately 1.1 million Americans have a heart attack each year.

Heart failure. Heart failure is the inability of the heart to pump blood efficiently. It affects 4.9 million Americans.

Arrhythmias. Arrhythmias are disturbances in the heart's rhythm. Atrial fibrillation—one of the most common arrhythmias—affects 2.2 million Americans.

In the United States, risk factors for CHD—such as smoking, high blood pressure, abnormal blood lipid levels, obesity, and diabetes—are so widespread that a survey of more than 90,000 adults found that only 18% had no risk factors for the disorder. Identifying and controlling risk factors for CHD can help prevent or delay the development and progression of the disease.

When preventive efforts are not enough, CHD and its complications can usually be managed through lifestyle measures, medications, revascularization procedures (angioplasty or bypass surgery), or a combination of all three. Medical advances have improved the management of angina as well as the likelihood of recovering from a heart attack. However, people with CHD should be aware that these advances often have their own risks, including side effects from medications and complications from surgical procedures.

The purpose of this White Paper is to provide people with sufficient knowledge about the prevention and treatment of CHD so that they can work closely and effectively with their doctors.

STRUCTURE OF THE HEART

The heart is composed almost entirely of muscle and contains four hollow chambers. The two upper chambers are the left atrium and the right atrium; the two lower chambers are the left ventricle and the right ventricle. Each heartbeat involves a muscular contraction that sends blood through the body's circulatory system. The left ventricle pumps oxygenated blood out of the heart via the aorta—the body's largest artery—which branches off into smaller arteries throughout the body. These arteries, in turn, divide into even smaller blood vessels, called arterioles, and eventually into capillaries, the microscopic blood vessels that deliver oxygen and nutrients to the cells and pick up carbon dioxide and other waste products from these cells.

After the deoxygenated blood passes through the capillaries, it enters tiny veins called venules and then travels back to the heart through progressively larger veins. When the blood reaches the heart, it enters the right atrium and then the right ventricle, which pumps the blood through the pulmonary arteries into the lungs. In the lungs, carbon dioxide in the blood is exchanged for fresh oxygen. The oxygenated blood then passes through the pulmonary veins into the left atrium, enters the left ventricle, and is pumped through the aorta to the rest of the body. This cycle is repeated about 100,000 times per day.

Like other tissues, the heart muscle needs a steady supply of oxygen-rich blood in order to function. Heart muscle cells do not extract oxygen and nutrients directly from the blood that continually fills the heart's chambers. Instead, the heart receives its blood supply from the coronary arteries, which emerge from the base of the aorta. The principal coronary arteries are the right coronary artery, left anterior descending artery, and left circumflex artery. All three arteries lie on the surface of the heart and branch off into smaller arteries. These branches, in turn, split into even smaller arteries (and eventually into capillaries) that extend deep into the heart muscle. The capillaries provide oxygen and nutrients to all portions of the heart and pick up waste products. The deoxygenated blood then passes through the coronary veins and into the right atrium.

How Coronary Heart Disease Leads To Angina

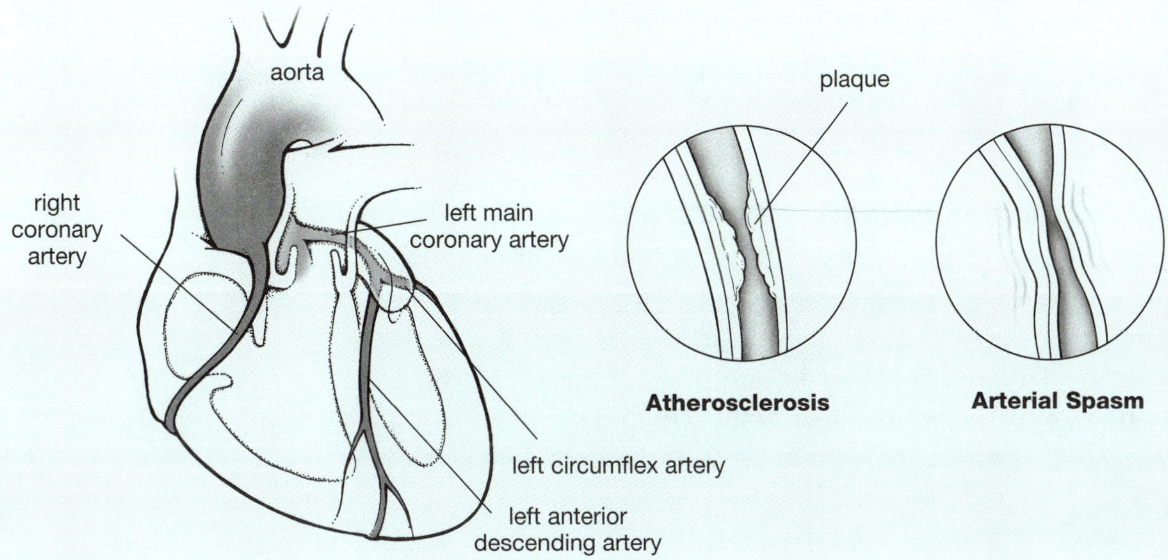

Coronary heart disease (CHD) is caused by the buildup of lesions, called atherosclerotic plaques, in the arteries supplying the heart. Like other organs, the heart needs a steady supply of oxygenated blood in order to function. But the heart cannot extract oxygen and nutrients directly from the blood that passes through its four inner chambers (the two atria on top and the two ventricles below); instead, heart cells receive their blood supply via the coronary arteries that branch off from the aorta (see the illustration above left). In people with CHD, atherosclerotic plaques narrow these arteries and impede blood flow to the heart muscle (see the illustration above center).

The first signs of atherosclerosis often appear in young individuals. Indeed, a significant number of men in their teens and 20s have early fatty streaks in the walls of their coronary arteries. But it usually takes several decades for plaques to grow large enough to cause symptoms. When coronary arteries become narrowed by 60% to 70%, blood flow to the heart may be insufficient during periods of physical exertion or emotional stress. The resulting deficiency of blood (ischemia) to the heart muscle typically causes chest pain known as angina. (However, up to 25% of patients with CHD do not experience angina, despite a shortage of blood to the heart; this condition is known as silent ischemia.)

Angina may also result from arterial spasm—a sudden contraction of the muscular layer encircling a coronary artery that narrows a portion of the artery (see the illustration above right). Interruption of blood flow through the artery results in a condition known as variant (or Prinzmetal's) angina, which differs from typical angina because it usually occurs while a person is at rest (generally between midnight and 8 A.M.) and does not follow a predictable pattern.

About two thirds of people with variant angina also have severe atherosclerosis in at least one coronary artery, and the spasms tend to occur close to the plaques. While typical angina usually subsides promptly with rest or medications such as nitrates, variant angina responds less well to these therapies. Calcium channel blockers appear to be more effective than beta-blockers when spasm is the primary cause of ischemia.

CAUSES OF CORONARY HEART DISEASE

The major underlying cause of CHD is atherosclerosis—the buildup of deposits called plaques within the walls of arteries. Plaques decrease the size of the lumen, the space through which blood flows in the arteries. When atherosclerosis develops in the coronary arteries, blood flow to the heart may be decreased (causing angina) or completely blocked (resulting in a heart attack).

Atherosclerosis is a multistep process. It begins with injury to the endothelium (the layer of cells that line the inside of arteries) and is exacerbated by the accumulation of oxidized low density lipoprotein (LDL) particles within the artery walls. High blood levels of LDL cholesterol and triglycerides, high blood pressure, and toxins from tobacco smoke help initiate and propagate this process.

Next, white blood cells called monocytes migrate to the intima (an area just below the endothelium), possibly in an attempt to repair the injury to the endothelium. In the intima, the monocytes are converted into macrophages, which act as scavengers that ingest oxidized LDL particles. As the macrophages take in more and more oxidized LDL particles, they undergo a second transformation—this time into cholesterol-laden foam cells.

The oxidized LDL particles cause further damage to the endothelium. This event attracts more monocytes, which enter the intima, are converted to macrophages, begin to consume oxidized LDL particles, and eventually become foam cells as well.

Damage to the endothelium also stimulates the growth of smooth muscle cells. These cells and the macrophages secrete collagen and other fibrous proteins. The result is a plaque composed of smooth muscle cells, fibrous proteins, and cholesterol-laden foam cells. The portion of the plaque that faces the bloodstream develops a fibrous cap, a firm shell containing calcium.

Angina occurs when plaque in a coronary artery grows large enough to hinder the flow of blood to the heart. Sometimes, the plaque's fibrous cap ruptures and a blood clot forms. This blood clot can completely block the coronary artery, causing a heart attack, or it may break loose and lodge within a smaller artery leading to the heart, also resulting in a heart attack.

SYMPTOMS AND COMPLICATIONS OF CORONARY HEART DISEASE

CHD can lead to a number of complications, including angina, heart attacks, heart failure, and arrhythmias.

Angina

Angina is pain or discomfort, usually in the chest, precipitated by myocardial ischemia—a shortage of blood and oxygen to the heart muscle due to partial blockage of a coronary artery. Angina occurs most often during physical activity, when the heart requires more oxygen but cannot get a sufficient supply because of the narrowing of one or more coronary arteries. Symptoms of angina usually occur when an artery is narrowed by at least 60% to 70%.

A sensation of pressure beneath the sternum (breastbone) is the most common symptom of angina, but some people experience feelings of tightness, squeezing, burning, aching, heaviness, or choking in this area. Angina can also produce pain in the left shoulder that radiates up to the neck and jaw, or pain in the inner part of the left arm that may travel down to the fingers. The intensity of the discomfort usually increases steadily, reaches a plateau, and gradually diminishes with rest—all within a few minutes. Rarely, the pain is sharp.

Women do not always experience angina in the same way as men. They are more likely than men to have angina when at rest or under emotional stress. In addition, they may feel angina as pain in the jaw or as heartburn. Other vague symptoms common in women include breathlessness, nausea, and fatigue, which can make diagnosis of the condition difficult.

Angina is often triggered by walking. The distance that can be walked without discomfort tends to vary somewhat from day to day, but most people can predict what level of exertion is likely to produce angina. Physical activity is more likely to bring on angina when undertaken early in the morning, after a meal, during cold weather, or when walking up an incline or into the wind. Activities involving use of the arms—such as shoveling, sweeping, scrubbing, or raking—may cause angina in some people. Sexual intercourse and bowel movements are other possible triggers. Anger, fear, anxiety, and excitement also can cause episodes of angina or reduce the amount of physical activity required to produce angina. The pain is usually promptly relieved by rest or by taking a nitrate medication.

Classification system. A system developed by the Canadian Cardiovascular Society categorizes the severity of angina into four classes and is widely used in the United States.

- **Class I.** Ordinary physical activity—such as walking or climbing stairs—does not cause angina. Angina only occurs with strenuous, rapid, or prolonged physical exertion during work or recreation.
- **Class II.** Associated with some limitation of ordinary activity. Angina occurs when walking or climbing stairs rapidly or when walking uphill. It also occurs when walking or climbing stairs after a meal, in cold or windy weather, when under emotional stress, or during the first few hours after awakening.

NEW RESEARCH

Asthma May Be Mistaken for Angina in Some People

Some people who come to the emergency department with chest pain may be having an attack of asthma rather than angina, according to Austrian researchers.

The researchers studied 41 people, age 30 to 81, who had experienced chest pain and had angina ruled out as the cause. None had been diagnosed with a lung disorder or coronary heart disease.

Tests of lung function revealed that four participants had chronic obstructive pulmonary disease (COPD). Of the remaining 37, 26 had decreased lung function after inhaling the drug methacholine (Provocholine), a trigger for asthma; 25 of the 26 developed symptoms of asthma such as shortness of breath and tightness or burning feelings in the chest. Twenty of them said that these were the same symptoms that brought them to the hospital.

According to the authors, about 1 in 10 people with chest pain who are referred for a heart evaluation do not have heart disease. When determining the cause of chest pain, doctors should also consider gastroesophageal reflux disease, nerve problems, and chest wall pain, the authors say.

EUROPEAN RESPIRATORY JOURNAL
Volume 21, page 473
March 2003

Walking more than two level blocks or climbing more than one flight of stairs at a normal pace brings on angina.

- **Class III.** Associated with marked limitations of ordinary physical activity. Angina occurs when walking one to two level blocks or climbing one flight of stairs at a normal pace.
- **Class IV.** Characterized by an inability to perform any physical activity without discomfort. Angina symptoms may be present even at rest.

Silent ischemia. Many people with CHD have myocardial ischemia without symptoms of angina. This condition is called silent ischemia. People with angina may have episodes of silent ischemia in addition to angina pain.

Stable angina. The most common type of angina is referred to as stable angina, because a predictable amount of activity or stress triggers an attack, the amount and duration of the pain are similar in each attack, and pain is promptly relieved by rest or a nitrate drug.

Unstable angina. Unstable angina, sometimes called crescendo angina, is a condition intermediate in severity between stable angina and a heart attack. In unstable angina, an increased demand for oxygen may not be responsible for the inadequate supply of oxygen to the heart. Instead, a blood clot or coronary artery spasm decreases the supply of oxygen. As the artery narrows, too little oxygen is delivered to the heart muscle and angina results.

Unstable angina has three major features. First, angina occurs at rest and usually lasts for longer than 20 minutes. Second, angina is severe enough to cause a marked limitation of ordinary activity (for example, pain when climbing one flight of stairs or walking two blocks at a normal pace). Third, the pattern of angina changes so that the pain is more frequent, lasts longer, and is brought on by less physical activity.

Unstable angina often requires treatment in a hospital. The risk of a heart attack or ventricular fibrillation (see pages 11–12) is increased in people with unstable angina because atherosclerotic plaque in the affected coronary artery can rupture and lead to a blood clot that may grow rapidly and cause complete blockage of the artery.

Heart Attack

Unlike angina, in which the coronary arteries become partially blocked, a heart attack occurs when one of the coronary arteries becomes completely blocked. Most often, the cause of the blockage is a blood clot that forms where a coronary artery is narrowed by atherosclerotic plaque that has ruptured. Many people who have heart attacks have a history of angina, and some experience more frequent or more severe angina pain in the days preceding the attack. Others may have ill-defined warning symptoms, such as increasing fatigue and shortness of breath. In many cases, however, a heart attack strikes suddenly and without any warning.

It is essential to get immediate medical help when symptoms suggest a heart attack. Nearly half of the deaths from heart attacks occur within the first hour, but the chances of survival are greatly improved in people who receive prompt medical attention. The following are warning signs of a heart attack:

- Uncomfortable pressure, fullness, squeezing, or pain in the center of the chest that lasts longer than 10 minutes;
- Pain spreading to the jaw, neck, shoulders, arms (especially the left arm), back, or upper abdomen; and
- Chest discomfort accompanied by light-headedness, sweating, nausea, shortness of breath, and/or fainting.

Not everyone experiences the same symptoms of a heart attack, and in some cases people have no symptoms at all. Men usually feel severe pain and pressure in the chest, while most women experience pain in the shoulder, upper back, neck, and jaw. Women are also more likely than men to have vague symptoms, such as mild chest pain, shortness of breath, dizziness, heartburn, or nausea. Unfortunately, the nonspecific nature of these symptoms may delay a trip to the hospital, interfere with diagnosis, and thus delay treatment. A study of about 6,000 men and women age 65 and older found that 22% had experienced a heart attack but were not aware of it. Another study of 43,000 heart attack patients found that a third did not have chest pain at the time of their heart attack.

Anyone experiencing symptoms that are suggestive of a heart attack and last longer than 10 minutes should seek immediate help by dialing 911 to call an ambulance. If the ambulance cannot arrive within 30 minutes, another person should drive the patient to the nearest emergency room. The person experiencing the heart attack symptoms should never drive himself or herself to the hospital, unless there is absolutely no other alternative. In addition, the person suffering symptoms should immediately chew a regular-dose aspirin to inhibit blood clotting. Emergency personnel must be told if an aspirin has been taken.

Serious complications can accompany or follow a heart attack. The ischemia associated with a heart attack results in death of heart muscle cells in the area supplied by the blocked artery. Loss of heart muscle can limit the heart's ability to pump blood efficiently.

NEW RESEARCH

Too Little, Too Much Sleep Tied to Heart Attacks

Women who get significantly less or significantly more than eight hours of sleep a night on average have an elevated risk of heart attacks and cardiac death, according to investigators from Boston.

The researchers obtained sleep data from 71,617 women, age 45 to 65, who did not have known CHD. Ten years later, compared with women who slept an average of eight hours a night, those who slept five or fewer hours a night had a 45% increased risk of experiencing a nonfatal heart attack or CHD-related death.

Diabetes, high blood pressure, and high cholesterol levels were more common among the women who slept the least. These factors may explain some of the increased risk of CHD in these women. Because the association persisted even after statistically adjusting for these and other CHD risk factors, however, sleep deprivation may have an independent effect on CHD risk.

Unexpectedly, women who got nine or more hours of sleep a night had a 38% increased risk of CHD compared with those who averaged eight hours of sleep. The reasons for this were unclear.

Adequate daily sleep "should not be considered a luxury," the authors conclude, "but an important component of a healthy lifestyle."

ARCHIVES OF INTERNAL MEDICINE
Volume 163, page 205
January 27, 2003

Sleep Apnea and Your Heart

Nighttime breathing disturbances may increase the risk of high blood pressure and heart problems.

Sleep apnea, characterized by repeated episodes of breathing cessation (apnea) during sleep, often causes daytime fatigue. But sleep apnea can also affect the heart and other parts of the cardiovascular system. For example, it increases the risk of high blood pressure, and several new studies have found associations between sleep apnea and atrial fibrillation, coronary heart disease (CHD), and heart failure.

What Is Sleep Apnea?

Sleep apnea results from a collapse and blockage of the upper airway during sleep (obstructive sleep apnea [OSA]), or a central nervous system abnormality that interferes with brain mechanisms that control breathing (central sleep apnea [CSA]). Risk factors for OSA include obesity, older age, cigarette smoking, weakness of the airway muscles, hypothyroidism (insufficient production of thyroid hormone), and a large neck. CSA, on the other hand, often results from a disease or injury of the brainstem but can also occur in people with heart failure.

Sleep apnea is more common in men, but women (particularly postmenopausal women) also suffer from the disorder. Previous epidemiological studies estimated that sleep apnea affects 2% of women and 4% of men in the United States, but a 2003 study in the *Journal of the American Medical Association* suggests that about 7% of the U.S. population may have sleep apnea. Most of these cases are OSA; CSA is rare in otherwise healthy people. Most people with OSA (95%) remain undiagnosed and untreated.

The first steps in treating OSA are lifestyle measures, such as losing weight, avoiding alcohol and sedatives at bedtime, quitting smoking, and sleeping on your side or in a more upright position. If these measures are not successful, a common treatment is continuous positive airway pressure (CPAP), which involves wearing a nasal mask that delivers a steady stream of pressurized air to keep the airways open. This therapy is effective in 80% to 90% of people.

There is no proven treatment for CSA at this time, although several therapies are being investigated.

High Blood Pressure

More than half of those with sleep apnea also have high blood pressure, and their blood pressure levels do not fall during sleep as occurs in most people. In fact, sleep apnea is an independent, treatable cause of high blood pressure. Sleep apnea likely leads to high blood pressure by causing a rapid rise in heart rate when breathing resumes. Some evidence suggests that periods of apnea and low blood oxygen levels, along with persistently high blood pressure, increase the risk of coronary heart disease (CHD). Both OSA and CSA can contribute to high blood pressure.

A 2003 study in *The Lancet* reported that CPAP was associated with a small but significant reduction in blood pressure in people with OSA. Researchers randomly assigned 118 men with OSA to either standard CPAP or CPAP at an air pressure that was too low to be therapeutic. One month later, patients receiving therapeutic CPAP had a 2.5 mm Hg reduction in mean blood pressure, compared with a 0.8 mm Hg increase in patients receiving subtherapeutic CPAP. The researchers estimate that this reduction in blood pressure translates to a 20% lower risk of stroke and a 15% lower risk of a coronary event, such as a heart attack.

Atrial Fibrillation

Sleep apnea can also affect atrial fibrillation, one of the most common heart rhythm abnormalities. In atrial fibrillation, the atria, or upper chambers of the heart, quiver rapidly and irregularly, rather than in a rhythmic pattern, and the ventricles begin to contract rapidly and irregularly as well. As a result, blood is not circulated efficiently to the body. Atrial fibrillation itself usually is not life-threatening, but it can lead to heart failure and increase the likelihood of blood clots in the heart. One of these blood

Poor pumping may lead to heart failure (see pages 10–11) or an insufficient supply of blood to other tissues, such as the brain. Ischemia can also damage the electrical system of the heart and lead to arrhythmias (see pages 11–12).

A severe form of heart failure, called cardiogenic shock, can occur when a heart attack damages more than 40% of the heart muscle. Untreated cardiogenic shock is fatal in 80% to 90% of cases;

clots could then travel to the brain and cause a stroke.

In a 2003 study reported in *Circulation*, OSA appeared to increase the risk of recurrence of atrial fibrillation. Researchers studied 39 people with atrial fibrillation and OSA; 27 of them either were not receiving CPAP treatment or were using the treatment incorrectly. A control group of 79 people had atrial fibrillation but had never been diagnosed with OSA. One year after successful treatment for atrial fibrillation, the condition recurred in 82% of the untreated or incorrectly treated OSA patients, 42% of the treated OSA patients, and 53% of the control group.

This study is the first to show that untreated or incorrectly treated OSA is associated with an increased risk of recurrence of atrial fibrillation. The researchers theorize that people with OSA may inhale more forcefully to overcome the airway obstruction. This action may raise blood pressure, lower the level of oxygen in the blood, and cause the walls of the heart to stretch—all of which can make a rhythm abnormality more likely. As a result, people with atrial fibrillation should be screened for OSA if they are obese, their spouses say they snore loudly or stop breathing during sleep, or they fall asleep during the daytime.

Coronary Heart Disease (CHD)

Several of the risk factors for OSA (such as obesity, older age, and cigarette smoking) also increase the risk of CHD. In fact, OSA is much more common in people who have CHD than in those who do not.

A 2003 study in the *American Journal of Respiratory and Critical Care Medicine* reported that OSA appears to increase the risk of cardiovascular disease fivefold. Researchers conducted sleep studies in 182 men (average age 47) without high blood pressure or other cardiovascular disease; 122 of the men had OSA and 60 did not. The men with OSA who had daytime sleepiness were offered treatment. Seven years later, one or more cardiovascular events (such as a heart attack, stroke, or diagnosis of hypertension or angina) had occurred in 37% of the men who had OSA, compared with 7% of the men who did not have OSA. Within the OSA group, cardiovascular events occurred in 57% of the men with untreated or incompletely treated OSA, but in only 7% of the men whose OSA was treated successfully.

Heart Failure

More than half of people with heart failure (an inability of the heart to pump blood efficiently) also have OSA or CSA. Both types of apnea appear to contribute to the progression of heart failure.

Studies strongly implicate OSA as a risk factor for heart failure; for example, one study of more than 6,000 adults reported that OSA more than doubled the risk of heart failure. During sleep, blood pressure and heart rate drop, which decreases the heart's workload. However, sleep apnea causes interruptions in breathing, which place stress on the heart. Over time, this repeated stress may cause the heart to enlarge and pump less efficiently, leading to heart failure.

A 2003 study in *The New England Journal of Medicine* suggests that treating OSA can improve heart failure. Twelve patients with both heart failure and OSA were treated with their usual drug therapy plus CPAP; 12 other patients with both conditions simply continued their drug therapy. After one month, the control group had no significant improvement in either OSA or heart function; however, the CPAP group had decreases in daytime blood pressure and heart rate, as well as improvements in heart function.

Two studies have reported that CSA is present in 33% and 40% of people with heart failure, respectively, a much higher percentage than in the general population.

Although CSA is often considered a symptom rather than a cause of heart failure, a 2003 study in *Circulation* suggests that CSA may contribute to the development of heart failure in susceptible people. Researchers conducted sleep studies in 47 people with left ventricular dysfunction (a precursor to heart failure). CSA was present in 55% of the patients, and 36% of them had severe CSA. The CSA patients also had more heart arrhythmias than the patients with normal breathing during sleep. The researchers say their findings suggest that CSA is a risk factor for heart failure.

treatment may reduce the risk of death to about 60%. In addition, the damaged portion of the heart may become so weak that the heart muscle ruptures, a condition that usually requires immediate open heart surgery to save the person's life. More commonly, the development of a bulge (aneurysm) in the heart wall at the site of the damaged muscle decreases the pumping efficiency of the heart.

The efficiency of the heart also may suffer from damage to small muscles that regulate the action of the mitral valve, one of the four valves that help control blood flow through the heart. In addition, blood clots may form in areas of the heart where muscle tissue has been damaged or has died. If pieces of these clots break off and travel through the body (such clots are called emboli), they can block blood vessels in the brain or elsewhere in the body, causing problems such as strokes, kidney damage, or gangrene. Finally, pericarditis, an inflammation of the membrane surrounding the outside of the heart, may occur after a heart attack and cause further pain.

Heart Failure

Heart failure is an impairment of the heart's pumping ability. The condition was formerly called congestive heart failure because it caused accumulation of fluid (congestion) in the lungs and other tissues. Now that medications are available to treat these symptoms, the term *congestive heart failure* is falling out of favor.

About 550,000 new cases of heart failure are diagnosed each year. The most common causes of heart failure are CHD, heart attacks, and high blood pressure (hypertension); other causes include heart valve abnormalities due to rheumatic fever, heart defects present at birth, and infection of the heart valves or heart muscle.

The symptoms of heart failure include fatigue, shortness of breath (dyspnea), fluid retention (edema), and excessive urination at night (nocturia). In most cases, symptoms are initially mild—for example, feeling overly tired after physical exertion—but eventually even slight activity becomes exhausting. In people with untreated heart failure, fluid settles in the lungs when lying down. This causes extreme shortness of breath and awakening at night (paroxysmal nocturnal dyspnea); sitting up may relieve these symptoms. Severe shortness of breath, often accompanied by wheezing, coughing, and blood-tinged phlegm, indicates pulmonary edema (marked buildup of fluid in the lungs), which generally requires immediate medical treatment. Older people with heart failure may also experience light-headedness or confusion.

The following system, developed by the New York Heart Association, is widely used to classify the severity of heart failure:

- **Class I.** Symptoms appear with greater than ordinary activity, but not with ordinary activity;
- **Class II.** Person is comfortable at rest but has some limitation of activity;
- **Class III.** Person is comfortable at rest but has marked limitation of activity; and

- **Class IV.** Discomfort occurs with any physical activity, and symptoms of heart failure may be present at rest.

Arrhythmias

A normal heartbeat begins with an electrical signal generated by cells in the upper right part of the heart—a region called the sinus node. The sinus node is the heart's natural pacemaker, telling the heart when to beat.

During normal activity, the sinus node sends an electrical signal 60 to 80 times a minute. The signal from the sinus node passes through the right and left atria, causing them to contract, and then pauses briefly in the atrioventricular (AV) node—a cluster of cells in the center of the heart. This delay allows the atria to pump blood into the ventricles just before the ventricles themselves contract. Finally, the signal travels through a network of pathways in the ventricles (His-Purkinje system) and stimulates the ventricles to contract and pump blood through the aorta to the rest of the body.

The various types of arrhythmias are distinguished by two features: their site of origin and their effect on heart rate. Arrhythmias can originate in the atria, the AV node, or the ventricles and can produce a heart rate that is either too slow (bradycardia) or too fast (tachycardia).

Atrial fibrillation. One of the most common abnormal rhythms originating in the atria is atrial fibrillation, in which electrical signals are initiated from the atrial muscle rather than from the sinus node. Instead of contracting in a regular pattern, the atria quiver (fibrillate) quickly and chaotically and the ventricles contract rapidly and irregularly as well. As a result, blood is not circulated efficiently to the rest of the body. The risk of atrial fibrillation is increased by age, cardiovascular disease (disease of the heart or circulatory system), heart valve abnormalities, or an overactive thyroid (hyperthyroidism).

Atrial fibrillation may cause weakness, light-headedness, shortness of breath, heart palpitations, and chest pain, although some people experience no symptoms. It can also lead to the formation of blood clots in the atria. These blood clots become dangerous when they loosen and form emboli that travel through the circulatory system. Emboli can block arteries supplying blood to vital organs. When they block an artery carrying blood to the brain, the result is a stroke.

Ventricular tachycardia and ventricular fibrillation. Arrhythmias that are initiated within the ventricles are potentially more serious than arrhythmias that begin in the atria. Ventricular arrhythmias,

NEW RESEARCH

Flu Shot Decreases Risk of Heart Attack, Stroke

An annual flu vaccine may reduce the risk of a heart attack or stroke, as well as of dying of any cause, according to a new study.

Researchers studied two groups of people over age 65: 140,055 adults in the 1998 to 1999 flu season, and 146,328 in the 1999 to 2000 flu season. In the earlier flu season, 56% of the participants received a flu shot, as did 60% of the participants in the later flu season. Adults who received a flu shot were 19% less likely to be hospitalized for heart disease during both seasons. The flu shot was also associated with a reduced risk during each season of being hospitalized for stroke by 20%, being hospitalized for flu or pneumonia by 30%, and dying of any cause by 49%.

Experts theorize that the flu may make heart attacks and strokes more likely by affecting blood clotting or blood vessel dilation, or by causing dehydration. It is also possible that those who get the vaccine engage in other healthy habits that lower their risk.

The flu vaccine was associated with similar benefits for healthy older adults as well as those with health problems, and the researchers stress the importance of the flu vaccine for all adults over the age of 65. In 2001, only 63% of American adults over age 65 received the flu vaccine.

THE NEW ENGLAND JOURNAL OF MEDICINE
Volume 348, page 1322
April 3, 2003

such as ventricular tachycardia and ventricular fibrillation, are often due to damage to the heart muscle. These rhythm disturbances can occur during a heart attack, when dying heart muscle releases cellular products that interfere with normal electrical activity in the heart. After a heart attack, ventricular arrhythmias can originate in the area where scar tissue forms.

Ventricular tachycardia is usually accompanied by severe symptoms, especially in those with significant heart damage. Inefficient pumping can result in light-headedness, severe weakness, fainting, heart failure with pulmonary edema, heart attack, stroke, and, in the worst-case scenario, cardiac arrest (sudden cessation of the heartbeat). Depending on how fast the heart rate is, people with ventricular tachycardia can survive for hours without treatment. In the case of ventricular fibrillation, however, the pumping action of the heart is totally lost, and death occurs in a few minutes without treatment.

Milder types of arrhythmias. These types of arrhythmias are usually due to problems with the AV node or the electrical system of the atria. People may experience palpitations (fluttering, racing, or skipped beats) with irregular or very rapid rhythms. Extreme bradycardia (fewer than 45 beats per minute) and tachycardia (more than 140 beats per minute at rest) can result in shortness of breath, light-headedness, and fainting. Angina or a heart attack may occur in people with tachycardia when the coronary arteries are unable to supply enough oxygen to meet the extra workload produced by a very rapid heart rate.

RISK FACTORS FOR CORONARY HEART DISEASE

The most important risk factors for CHD are cigarette smoking, high blood pressure, abnormal blood lipid levels, diabetes, family history of premature CHD events, and older age. Risk factors for CHD can be divided into two categories: those that cannot be modified and those that can. The more risk factors a person has, the greater the chance of developing CHD.

Risk Factors That Cannot Be Modified

The presence of these nonmodifiable risk factors should alert those affected to consider taking preventive steps against CHD.

Age. The risk of CHD increases with age, especially in men age 45 and older and women age 55 and older. More than half of people who have a heart attack—and four out of five who die of a heart attack—are over age 65.

Gender. CHD is more common in young men than in young women. After menopause, however, when low levels of estrogen lead to an increase in LDL cholesterol and a drop in high density lipoprotein (HDL) cholesterol, women's risk of CHD begins to increase. By around age 75, a woman's CHD risk is equal to that of a man's. In fact, CHD is the major cause of death in postmenopausal women. The risk of CHD in women who undergo menopause before age 40 (because of surgical removal of the ovaries or spontaneous ovarian failure) is similar to that of postmenopausal women.

Heredity. People are at increased risk for CHD if they have a male first-degree relative (a father or brother) who has experienced a CHD event (such as a heart attack or CHD-related death) before age 55 or a female first-degree relative (a mother or sister) who has had a CHD event before age 65.

Diabetes. People with diabetes are two to five times more likely to develop CHD than people without diabetes. One reason is that elevated triglycerides, low HDL cholesterol, high blood pressure, and obesity, all of which are risk factors for CHD, are more common in people with diabetes. In addition, diabetes itself imparts other, unknown effects that increase the risk of CHD. For example, young women with diabetes lose the protection that other premenopausal women have against CHD; in fact, these women have the same risk of CHD as men.

Individuals with pre-diabetes (a condition in which blood glucose levels are higher than normal but not quite in the diabetic range) are also at increased risk for CHD. Pre-diabetes is diagnosed when blood glucose levels are between 110 and 125 mg/dL on a fasting blood glucose test or between 140 and 199 mg/dL on an oral glucose tolerance test.

Some studies suggest that careful control of blood glucose levels with diet and medication may help reduce the increased risk of CHD associated with diabetes. Thus, it is particularly important for people with diabetes or pre-diabetes to control other risk factors for CHD, such as smoking, abnormal blood lipid levels, and high blood pressure.

Cerebrovascular disease. CHD is the most likely cause of death in people with cerebrovascular disease (blockage of an artery that supplies blood to the brain). This is because people with evidence of blockage in these arteries invariably have blockages in the coronary arteries as well.

Peripheral vascular disease. For the same reason, CHD is also the most likely cause of death in people with peripheral vascular

NEW RESEARCH

Most CHD Patients Have Traditional Risk Factors

For many years, experts have said that only 50% of people with CHD have one of the four traditional CHD risk factors: high blood pressure, high cholesterol, diabetes, and smoking. Now, evidence shows that over 80% of people with CHD have at least one of these factors.

This conclusion was based on data from 14 published clinical trials that included 122,458 people who had heart attacks or unstable angina or were about to undergo angioplasty. Nearly 85% of women had at least one of the traditional risk factors, as did 81% of men. About 90% of people with CHD age 45 or younger had one or more of the factors, most often smoking.

A related study found that roughly 90% of healthy people who eventually die of CHD or have a nonfatal heart attack have at least one of these four major risk factors. The study involved 386,915 men and women, age 18 to 59, who were followed for 21 to 30 years.

According to an accompanying editorial, doctors and patients should "redouble efforts" to control traditional CHD risk factors.

JOURNAL OF THE AMERICAN MEDICAL ASSOCIATION
Volume 290, pages 891, 898, and 947
August 20, 2003

Many Tools for Smokers Who Want To Quit

Are you having trouble quitting smoking? Join a counseling group or try one of the many smoking-cessation products on the market.

Despite nearly 40 years of public health warnings about the dangers of tobacco, about a quarter of Americans still smoke. Cigarette smoking results in 440,000 premature deaths each year in the United States, and at least 179,000 of these are the direct result of heart attacks or strokes. Nonetheless, the damage caused by years of smoking often can be halted or partially reversed by quitting. And as new smoking-cessation products hit the market, smokers have a variety of options to help them kick the habit.

How Smoking Affects the Heart, Blood, and Arteries

Smoking's most direct effect is on the lungs, but it also increases the chances of developing and dying of coronary heart disease. Here's how:

- Smoking increases low density lipoprotein (LDL, or "bad") cholesterol levels and decreases high density lipoprotein (HDL, or "good") cholesterol levels.
- Cigarette smoke damages the inner walls of arteries, which initiates the process of atherosclerosis.
- Smoking also contributes to the progression of atherosclerosis by increasing the accumulation of LDL particles and monocytes (a type of white blood cell) in the artery walls.
- Smoking decreases the flexibility of arteries.
- Lastly, cigarette smoking causes blood to clot more easily.

Quitting Smoking

Because only about 8% of people who try to quit smoking are able to do so on their own, you can increase your chances of success by talking to your doctor about smoking cessation. Your doctor may be able to provide literature, advice, support, and medication to help you quit; he or she may also refer you to a health care professional who specializes in counseling for smoking cessation.

Counseling. Attending individual or group counseling sessions can increase your chances of success, and the more sessions you attend, the greater the likelihood of quitting. At these sessions, you will learn coping skills, relapse prevention, and stress management. The sessions also provide social support and encouragement.

Nicotine replacement therapy. Because nicotine is addictive, smoking cessation often leads to nicotine withdrawal, which can cause irritability, restlessness, food cravings, anxiety, and other symptoms. To help reduce these effects and control cravings for nicotine, your doctor may recommend or prescribe some form of nicotine replacement therapy—either gum, a skin patch, a nasal spray, an inhaler, or a lozenge. Using any of these products and gradually tapering the dosage doubles your chances of quitting successfully. You should start nicotine replacement on the day that you quit smoking.

Gum. Nicotine polacrilex gum (Nicorette) is available over the counter. The gum should be chewed only once or twice every few minutes and remain between your cheek and gum the rest of the time. Side effects, including nausea and indigestion, usually result from chewing the gum too much and swallowing large amounts of nicotine.

Skin patch. A nicotine patch may be easier and more convenient to use. Patches are available over the counter (Nicoderm CQ, Nicotrol) or by prescription (Habitrol). The patch should be changed daily. If it causes difficulty sleeping, try taking it off before going to bed. Also, do not smoke while on the patch. Smoking not only greatly reduces your chances of quitting but also can cause uncomfortably high blood levels of nicotine.

Nasal spray. Nicotine nasal spray

disease (blockage of the arteries that supply the extremities, most often the legs). Reduced blood pressure at the ankles or painful cramping in the legs upon exertion are signs of peripheral vascular disease.

Aortic valve sclerosis. The aortic valve controls the flow of blood from the left ventricle to the aorta. Aortic valve sclerosis is the hardening and thickening of this valve. In a study of nearly 6,000 adults age 65 or older, aortic valve sclerosis was associated with a 50% increased risk of a heart attack or CHD-related death. This is because

(Nicotrol NS) is available by prescription only. Your doctor can help you determine the exact timing and dose to use, but you should initially use no more than 80 sprays (40 in each nostril) daily. Side effects include nasal irritation, runny nose, throat irritation, and nausea.

Inhaler. Also available by prescription is a nicotine inhalation system (Nicotrol Inhaler). Patients typically begin with 6 to 16 inhaler cartridges per day and gradually taper the dose over a maximum of six months. Irritation of the mouth or throat is a potential adverse effect.

Lozenge. Nicotine lozenges (Commit Lozenges) are available over the counter. Smokers who habitually have their first cigarette within 30 minutes of waking should use the 4-mg lozenges; others should use the 2-mg version. You should use a lozenge every one to two hours (but no more than 20 per day) for the first 6 weeks of the 12-week program. After 6 weeks, use a lozenge every two to four hours, and then taper down to a lozenge every four to eight hours for weeks 10 through 12. Side effects may include nausea, hiccups, and heartburn.

Bupropion. Bupropion (Zyban) is a prescription medication for smoking cessation that contains no nicotine; it helps reduce cravings and withdrawal symptoms in some people. Researchers believe that the drug disrupts the pleasurable feelings that cigarette smoking typically produces in the brain. (Bupropion is also sold as an antidepressant called Wellbutrin and can be a good choice for people who have a mood disorder that could make smoking cessation more difficult.) People with a history of seizures, an eating disorder, or uncontrolled high blood pressure should not take bupropion. Side effects include trouble sleeping and dry mouth.

Combination therapy. The combination of counseling, nicotine replacement therapy, and bupropion provides the highest chance of success. In one study, people who used all three therapies at once had a 35% success rate.

Tips for Quitting

Quitting smoking can be difficult, and you may need to make numerous attempts before you are successful. If you have tried to quit before without long-lasting success, analyze what helped and what hindered you, and adjust your strategy accordingly.

Here are some tips used by successful quitters:

- Pick a quit date that has significant meaning—like New Year's Day or a birthday.
- Ask for support from family, friends, and coworkers. If any of them smoke, ask them not to smoke around you.
- Determine what events, situations, and other factors are cues to your smoking, and figure out ways to avoid them. For example, throw out ashtrays and lighters. If you always have a cigarette at a certain point during your drive home from work, try taking a different route. If you are used to having a cigarette with coffee after dinner, skip the coffee and do something else to distract yourself.
- Experts recommend that you avoid alcohol, or at least severely limit your intake, for the first three months after you quit. Alcohol can act as a trigger for smoking and also reduces your chances of success by decreasing inhibitions.
- Some people find that deep breathing, drinking lots of liquids (preferably water, rather than soft drinks, coffee, or tea), and exercising help them deal more successfully with cravings.
- If you are concerned about weight gain after smoking cessation, remember that people usually gain fewer than 10 lbs. after they quit. Furthermore, such weight gain has a much smaller impact on your health than does smoking.

aortic valve sclerosis results from the same process that causes atherosclerosis in the coronary arteries.

Blood-clotting factors. Formation of a blood clot within an artery is the final step in the atherosclerotic process that results in a heart attack. Efforts to find a consistent clotting abnormality in people prone to heart attacks have been unsuccessful. A number of studies have found an association between increased heart attack risk and elevated blood levels of fibrinogen or factor VII (two clotting proteins) or an over-responsiveness of platelets (cells involved in blood clotting) to certain stimuli. Elevated levels of plasminogen activator inhibitor (PAI-1; a substance that inhibits the breakdown of blood clots) also are associated with an increased risk of cardiovascular diseases like heart attack and stroke.

A variation in phospholipase A2 (PLA2), a protein involved in platelet aggregation, was the first inherited platelet risk factor to be identified for heart disease. A study conducted by a team of Johns Hopkins researchers found that heart attacks occurred more often in people who had the PLA2 variation than in those who did not.

Risk Factors That Can Be Modified

It is important to control or eliminate as many of these modifiable risk factors as possible.

Cigarette smoking. Cigarette smoking is a dangerous risk factor for CHD, as well as for lung cancer and many other disorders. Fortunately, much can be gained by stopping smoking. Even in people who have smoked for many years, the risk of a CHD event (such as a heart attack) returns to that of nonsmokers within five years of quitting. For help on quitting smoking, see the feature on pages 14–15.

High blood pressure. High blood pressure (hypertension) causes the left ventricle to enlarge and require more blood. At the same time, it increases the rate of atherosclerosis, thus limiting the heart's blood supply.

In its newest guidelines, the National Heart, Lung, and Blood Institute of the National Institutes of Health defines normal blood pressure as a systolic blood pressure of less than 120 mm Hg and a diastolic blood pressure of less than 80 mm Hg. Systolic blood pressure is the upper number in a blood pressure reading and represents pressure in the arteries while the heart is pumping blood to the rest of the body; diastolic blood pressure is the lower number and represents pressure in the arteries while the heart relaxes between beats.

People with a systolic blood pressure of 120 to 139 mm Hg or a diastolic blood pressure of 80 to 89 mm Hg are considered to have prehypertension. These individuals are more likely to develop high blood pressure and have a greater risk of cardiovascular events (for example, heart attacks and strokes) than those with lower blood pressures. High blood pressure is defined as a systolic blood pressure of 140 mm Hg or more or a diastolic blood pressure of 90 mm Hg or more. Lowering blood pressure in people with prehypertension or high blood pressure reduces the likelihood of a heart attack, lowers the risk of heart failure and stroke, and slows the progression of kidney disease.

For many years experts thought that both systolic and diastolic blood pressures, or at least diastolic pressure, had to be elevated to increase the risk of CHD. Now studies have demonstrated that elevated systolic blood pressure alone (called isolated systolic hypertension) is also risky. The incidence of isolated systolic hypertension increases with age and is the most common form of high blood pressure in the elderly. In one study, lowering blood pressure with medication in people with isolated systolic hypertension decreased the frequency of fatal and nonfatal heart attacks by 27%.

Abnormal levels of blood lipids and lipoproteins. Cholesterol and triglycerides are lipids that are carried through the bloodstream on proteins called lipoproteins. Cholesterol is transported on LDL or HDL; triglycerides are primarily carried on very low density lipoprotein (VLDL). Increased levels of total cholesterol, LDL cholesterol, and triglycerides and decreased levels of HDL cholesterol are associated with an elevated risk of CHD. To monitor CHD risk, all people over age 20 should have a blood test called a lipid profile at least every five years. The lipid profile determines the amount of total cholesterol, LDL cholesterol, HDL cholesterol, and triglycerides in the blood.

Increased total and LDL cholesterol levels boost the risk of CHD by increasing the amount of cholesterol deposited within the walls of the arteries. The National Cholesterol Education Program (NCEP) recommends that total cholesterol levels be kept below 200 mg/dL to reduce the risk of CHD. The target for LDL cholesterol depends on how many of the following risk factors a person has:

- cigarette smoking;
- high blood pressure (140/90 mm Hg or higher, or taking blood pressure-lowering medication);
- HDL cholesterol below 40 mg/dL;
- family history of a premature CHD event (under 55 years old in men, under 65 in women) in a first-degree relative; and
- older age (45 years or over in men, 55 or older in women).

For people with none or one of these risk factors, LDL cholesterol should be less than 160 mg/dL. In individuals with two or more of these risk factors, LDL cholesterol should be kept below 130 mg/dL. In all people with known cardiovascular disease (for example, CHD, stroke, or peripheral vascular disease) or diabetes, the NCEP guidelines state that LDL cholesterol should be lowered to less than 100 mg/dL.

NEW RESEARCH

Cholesterol Control Not Improving

Despite an increase in the number of prescriptions for cholesterol-lowering medications in recent years, average total cholesterol levels in the U.S. population are not decreasing, investigators from the Centers for Disease Control and Prevention report.

Between 1988 and 1994, average total cholesterol levels were 205 mg/dL, according to a previous study of 15,719 adult Americans. In the current report, the average total cholesterol level of 4,148 adults from 1999 to 2000 was 203 mg/dL, a statistically nonsignificant decrease from the earlier study. There were, however, significant reductions in cholesterol levels between the first and second studies in men age 75 and older, Mexican-American women, and black men.

These findings represent a significant shift from earlier years: Average total cholesterol levels fell 8 mg/dL when values from 1976 to 1980 were compared with those from 1988 to 1991.

The investigators also reported that in adults who had high cholesterol or were taking medication for the condition, only 35% were aware of their high cholesterol, 12% were being treated for it, and 5% were being successfully treated (i.e., had a total cholesterol level below 200 mg/dL).

The investigators conclude that "renewed efforts are necessary to lower total cholesterol concentrations in the U.S. population."

CIRCULATION
Volume 107, page 2185
May 6, 2003

A low HDL cholesterol level (less than 40 mg/dL) is considered a risk factor for CHD. In fact, recent research suggests that a total blood cholesterol level below 200 mg/dL—the level considered desirable—may still be associated with an increased CHD risk if HDL cholesterol levels are below 40 mg/dL, particularly in women. A high level of HDL cholesterol (60 mg/dL or higher), however, is considered protective against CHD and cancels out the effects of one other CHD risk factor when determining the total number of risk factors. HDL protects against CHD by transporting cholesterol from plaques within the walls of the arteries to the liver.

Triglyceride levels above 150 mg/dL are considered undesirable, but it has been difficult to determine whether high triglyceride levels directly raise the risk of CHD, since elevated triglycerides are frequently accompanied by low HDL cholesterol levels. But the latest research indicates that high triglyceride levels are a risk factor even when HDL cholesterol levels are normal.

The CHD risk of elevated triglycerides is especially great when combined with low levels of HDL cholesterol and small, dense LDL particles (see below). This pattern of risk factors is common in people who are obese or have diabetes or pre-diabetes. High triglyceride levels also impart high risk when associated with a high ratio of LDL to HDL cholesterol or the presence of familial combined hyperlipidemia or dysbetalipoproteinemia. These two disorders, which are caused by defective genes, result in high blood cholesterol, high blood triglycerides, or both.

Elevated triglyceride levels likely increase CHD risk by interfering with the normal widening of coronary arteries that occurs, for example, during physical exertion, and by increasing the risk of blood clots. Lowering triglycerides with weight loss, control of diabetes (if present), and lipid-lowering medications (when necessary) may raise HDL cholesterol levels and reduce the risk of CHD.

Size and density of LDL particles can affect CHD risk as well. LDL particles vary in size and density in a way that produces two patterns: A and B. People with pattern A have mostly large LDL particles, while people with pattern B have a predominance of small, dense particles. Pattern B patients have a higher risk of CHD than pattern A patients.

Men are more likely than women to have pattern B, which may be genetic or develop as a result of high triglyceride levels or diabetes. Smaller LDL particles increase the risk of CHD because they enter the walls of arteries more easily and are more prone to oxidation than are larger LDL particles. However, the presence of mostly

Evaluating Blood Levels Of Lipids and Lipoproteins

Everyone age 20 and over should have a blood test called a lipid profile at least once every five years to help determine their risk of coronary heart disease (CHD). The test measures the blood levels of total cholesterol, low density lipoprotein (LDL) cholesterol, high density lipoprotein (HDL) cholesterol, and triglycerides in the blood.

The table below shows the risk classifications for the blood lipids and lipoproteins measured in a lipid profile.

	Desirable	**Borderline**	**Increased Risk**
Total cholesterol	<200 mg/dL	200–239 mg/dL	≥240 mg/dL
LDL cholesterol	100-129 mg/dL*	130–159 mg/dL	≥160 mg/dL
HDL cholesterol	≥60 mg/dL	40–59 mg/dL	<40 mg/dL
Triglycerides	<150 mg/dL	150–199 mg/dL	≥200 mg/dL

*Optimal: <100 mg/dL.

small LDL particles is often associated with higher triglyceride levels and lower HDL cholesterol levels, a combination that may have a more important effect on CHD risk than particle size alone.

High levels of lipoprotein(a), also known as Lp(a), are another risk factor for CHD. Lp(a) is a lipoprotein with a structure similar to LDL but has on its surface another protein called apo (a) that resembles the blood protein plasminogen. Plasminogen is converted into the enzyme plasmin, which plays a role in dissolving blood clots in the arteries by breaking down fibrin, a major component of blood clots.

Two explanations have been proposed for why Lp(a) increases the risk of CHD. First, because of its similarity to plasminogen, Lp(a) might interfere with the conversion of plasminogen to plasmin, thus encouraging blood clots to persist. Second, like LDL, Lp(a) can be deposited within the walls of arteries and contribute to plaque formation. Unfortunately, Lp(a) levels are difficult to lower, though modest reductions may be achieved with high doses of niacin in some people and with hormone replacement therapy in postmenopausal women.

Obesity. Being overweight or obese increases the risk of CHD. Federal guidelines issued jointly by the National Heart, Lung, and Blood Institute and the National Institute of Diabetes and Digestive and Kidney Diseases recommend using body mass index (BMI) to determine who is overweight or obese. BMI is calculated by multiplying weight in pounds by 704 and dividing the result by the square of height in inches. Overweight is defined as a BMI of 25 to 29.9, and obesity as a BMI of 30 or over. Therefore, someone who is five feet ten inches tall is overweight at 174 lbs. and obese at 209 lbs.; someone five feet four inches tall is overweight at 145 lbs. and obese at 174 lbs.

Waist circumference is another method of measuring obesity and evaluating CHD risk. The adverse effects of obesity depend not only on the total amount of excess body fat but also on how it is distributed on the body. Abdominal obesity is particularly dangerous because it leads to insulin resistance (the reduced ability of the body to respond to insulin, a hormone that regulates blood glucose levels). Insulin resistance leads to elevated blood levels of insulin, which in turn are associated with high triglyceride levels, low levels of HDL cholesterol, high blood pressure, and increased CHD risk.

To measure waist circumference, place a tape measure around the waist, level with the top of the hip bones; the tape measure should feel snug without compressing the skin. Measure after exhaling normally. A waist circumference of greater than 40 inches in men or 35 inches in women indicates abdominal obesity and a heightened CHD risk.

Metabolic syndrome. A person is considered to have metabolic syndrome if he or she has at least three of the following five findings:

- abdominal obesity (a waist circumference greater than 40 inches in men or 35 inches in women);
- triglyceride levels of 150 mg/dL or greater;
- HDL cholesterol levels of less than 40 mg/dL in men or 50 mg/dL in women;
- blood pressures of 130/85 mm Hg or higher, or taking a blood pressure-lowering medication; and
- fasting blood glucose levels of 110 mg/dL or greater.

Nearly 50% of Americans over age 50 have metabolic syndrome, and the condition increases their risk of CHD, diabetes, and stroke. Metabolic syndrome can be treated with lifestyle measures, such as weight loss, physical activity, a fiber-rich diet, and smoking cessation, as well as with medications to improve lipid levels, lower blood pressure, and control blood glucose levels.

Physical inactivity. A large body of research shows that regular physical activity and physical fitness help prevent a first heart attack, and the American Heart Association cites physical inactivity as an important risk factor for CHD.

Regular exercise helps to control weight, lower blood pressure, and improve blood lipid levels. After a heart attack, exercise is an important component of a cardiac rehabilitation program because it significantly decreases the risk of recurrent CHD events.

Stress. Over the past 30 years, studies have shown a relationship between mental stress and various aspects of CHD. Physiological responses to stress include the release of epinephrine (adrenaline) and other hormones that speed heart rate, raise blood pressure, and may cause a spasm in the coronary arteries. If the coronary arteries are already narrowed by the buildup of plaque, a spasm could lead to angina or a heart attack. Nonetheless, stress is not generally accepted as a risk factor for CHD, partly because it is difficult to quantify the amount of stress in an individual's life.

Homocysteine. The amino acid homocysteine may increase the risk of CHD, as well as stroke and peripheral vascular disease. Experts are uncertain how homocysteine adversely affects the arteries, but high levels may promote atherosclerosis by damaging the endothelium and stimulating the growth of smooth muscle cells.

C-reactive protein (CRP). This protein is produced by the liver in response to tissue inflammation or infection, and elevated levels predict heart attacks and strokes many years before they occur. People with even small elevations of CRP appear to be at increased risk for CHD and its complications, regardless of their age, gender, general health, or the presence of other CHD risk factors. It is not known whether reducing CRP levels reduces the risk of CHD.

DIAGNOSIS OF CORONARY HEART DISEASE AND ITS COMPLICATIONS

Angina is suspected when a patient complains of chest pain. Tests such as an electrocardiogram (ECG or EKG), exercise stress test, and coronary angiography are then performed to confirm the presence of CHD and to help identify which coronary arteries are affected.

When people experience symptoms of a heart attack, the diagnosis usually can be confirmed by performing an ECG and measuring blood levels of certain proteins—creatine kinase, creatine kinase-MB, troponin, and myoglobin—that are released from damaged heart muscle.

If a doctor suspects heart failure based on the presence of fatigue, shortness of breath on exertion, and abnormal findings on a physical examination, commonly performed tests include a chest x-ray, ECG, and echocardiography. In the case of arrhythmias, electrophysiology studies may be needed in addition to an ECG.

NEW RESEARCH

Metabolic Syndrome Increases Risk of Heart Attack, Diabetes

Men with metabolic syndrome have a significantly elevated risk of having a heart attack or developing diabetes, according to a study of Scottish men.

The investigators identified the presence of metabolic syndrome in 6,447 men with moderately high levels of LDL cholesterol who had never had a heart attack or diabetes. Men were considered to have metabolic syndrome if they had at least three of these factors: high triglycerides, high blood pressure, low HDL cholesterol, elevated fasting blood glucose, or obesity.

After nearly five years, men with metabolic syndrome at the onset of the study were almost two times more likely to have a nonfatal heart attack or die of CHD than men without metabolic syndrome. The syndrome was also linked to a 3½-fold increased risk of diabetes. The men were much more likely to have a CHD event or develop diabetes if they had four or five factors for metabolic syndrome.

Using these five factors to diagnose metabolic syndrome "will help identify individuals who may receive particular benefit from lifestyle measures to prevent CHD and diabetes," the researchers conclude.

CIRCULATION
Volume 108, page 414
July 29, 2003

Electrocardiogram (ECG or EKG)

An ECG uses small metal sensors (electrodes) that are applied to the skin of the chest, arms, and legs to detect and record electrical signals from the heart. The test is especially valuable in detecting abnormal heart rhythms and new heart attacks; it may also indicate areas of heart muscle damaged from previous heart attacks. An ECG can also be used to detect thickening of the wall of the left ventricle and defects in the conduction of electrical impulses from the atria to the ventricles.

A normal resting ECG does not eliminate the possibility of myocardial ischemia, which may occur and cause chest pain only during increased physical activity. Silent ischemia can be detected using a Holter monitor (also called an ambulatory electrocardiogram), which records the heart's electrical activity over a 24-hour period. Two or more electrodes are placed on the chest and attached to a small, portable tape recorder that is worn on a belt around the waist. The 24-hour tape is then analyzed using a computer program to detect rhythm disturbances as well as abnormalities due to myocardial ischemia.

Holter monitoring is also useful in evaluating people with unexplained fainting or palpitations and in determining the effectiveness of antiarrhythmic drugs.

Exercise Stress Test

A standard exercise stress test uses an ECG to record the electrical impulses coming from the heart during exercise. The electrical signal often changes when the heart is not receiving enough blood and oxygen during physical activity.

In people who have chest pain or are at risk for CHD, an exercise stress test can be used to detect the presence of CHD. The test may also be performed to assess the safety and appropriate level of exercise for people beginning an exercise program after a heart attack or bypass surgery and to evaluate the effectiveness of certain treatments (such as those for arrhythmias).

The stress test involves walking on a treadmill or pedaling a stationary bicycle. The speed and incline of the treadmill or the resistance of the bicycle are gradually increased until the person reaches his or her target heart rate (at least 85% of maximal heart rate). The test may be stopped early if the person becomes fatigued or experiences symptoms such as chest pain, shortness of breath, dizziness, or an irregular heartbeat.

An exercise stress test is not always accurate in detecting the presence of CHD. In young women and other people at low risk for CHD, the test may be abnormal even though the coronary arteries are not blocked. The test is also associated with a very small risk of heart attack or cardiac arrest, but patients are carefully monitored during the test and treated right away if any serious complications occur.

Nuclear Medicine Stress Test

A nuclear medicine stress test is sometimes performed when a standard exercise stress test shows no clear abnormalities, but the person has symptoms that suggest angina. The test is similar to a standard stress test, but once the target heart rate is reached a radioactive substance—usually thallium—is injected into a vein in the arm. In those who cannot exercise, the radioactive substance is injected after the administration of dobutamine, a drug that simulates the effects of exercise on the heart.

Once injected, the radioactive substance travels through the bloodstream to the heart and is detected with a special camera. Heart muscle that receives blood from narrowed coronary arteries will have less radioactivity than heart muscle fed by healthy coronary arteries. To determine more precisely why certain areas of the heart are not getting enough blood, the amount of radioactivity in the heart may be remeasured when the heart is at rest on the same or next day.

A nuclear medicine stress test is more accurate than a standard exercise stress test. It detects CHD in about 20% of people whose resting and exercise ECGs are normal despite narrowing of their coronary arteries. As with a regular exercise stress test, there is a very small risk of a heart attack or cardiac arrest. The amount of radioactivity used is similar to that from an x-ray and is not considered dangerous. Side effects from dobutamine include headache, dizziness, chest discomfort, and nausea and vomiting.

Echocardiography

Echocardiography uses ultrasonic waves to determine the motion and ejection fraction of the left ventricle and to identify the presence of ventricular aneurysms and regions of abnormal heart function. (The ejection fraction is the amount of the blood in the left ventricle that is pumped out with each contraction. In a healthy individual, the ejection fraction ranges from 50% to 65%.) The procedure may also be used to detect defects in the walls dividing the chambers of the heart, valve disease, and blood clots within the chambers.

NEW RESEARCH

Fitness During Stress Test Good Predictor of CHD in Women

Doctors often use electrocardiogram (ECG) changes during an exercise stress test to predict the risk of a CHD event, but another factor measured by a stress test—exercise fitness—may be a better predictor of CHD risk in women without CHD symptoms.

The study included 2,994 women without CHD, age 30 to 80, who had an exercise stress test between 1972 and 1976. In addition to an ECG to detect decreased blood flow to the heart, researchers studied two measures of fitness: peak exercise capacity (the length of time the women could exercise) and heart rate recovery (peak heart rate minus heart rate two minutes after stopping exercise).

While ECG indicators of reduced blood flow to the heart (a significant predictor of CHD in men) did not predict the risk of cardiovascular death over the next 20 years, peak exercise capacity and heart rate recovery were significant predictors in these women. Women in the lower half of the group on measures of both exercise capacity and heart rate recovery were 3½ times more likely to die of cardiovascular disease than those in the top half on both measures.

These results strongly suggest that women may lower their risk of CHD by improving their physical fitness.

JOURNAL OF THE AMERICAN MEDICAL ASSOCIATION
Volume 290, page 1600
September 24, 2003

Boosting HDL Cholesterol Levels Without Drugs

You can make numerous lifestyle changes to increase your "good" cholesterol.

Lowering low density lipoprotein (LDL, or "bad") cholesterol levels is an important goal in preventing and managing coronary heart disease (CHD), but so is raising high density lipoprotein (HDL, or "good") cholesterol levels. Since the 1950s, researchers have known that high levels of HDL cholesterol decrease the risk of CHD and that low levels increase the risk. People with HDL cholesterol levels lower than 40 mg/dL have a significantly elevated risk of heart attacks and strokes. About 30% of people with CHD have low HDL cholesterol levels but normal levels of LDL cholesterol.

Data from recent drug studies show that raising low HDL cholesterol levels can decrease the rate of CHD events. In one study of more than 2,500 men with known CHD and normal LDL cholesterol but low HDL cholesterol levels, the medication gemfibrozil (Lopid) increased HDL cholesterol levels by 6% and the rate of CHD events dropped 22% with no significant decrease in LDL cholesterol. (But in a recent analysis of the results, researchers found that the incidence of CHD events was reduced only in those with diabetes or insulin resistance. No significant benefit of gemfibrozil treatment was seen in the other study participants.) In another study of men at high risk for CHD events, gemfibrozil raised HDL cholesterol levels by 11% while lowering the rate of CHD events by 34%. In this study, too, the benefit was particularly striking in those with diabetes.

These trials highlight the benefit of increasing low HDL cholesterol levels. In fact, increasing HDL cholesterol may be as important as decreasing LDL cholesterol for avoiding heart attacks and strokes.

Even though several medications, including gemfibrozil, fenofibrate (Lofibra, Tricor), statins, and niacin, can increase HDL cholesterol levels, four lifestyle measures—smoking cessation, exercise, weight loss, and dietary changes—may improve HDL cholesterol and should be undertaken whether or not any medications are used. Moderate alcohol intake also raises HDL cholesterol, but lifelong nondrinkers should not start drinking alcohol to improve their HDL levels. Estrogen replacement in postmenopausal women raises HDL cholesterol levels significantly, but the Women's Health Initiative study found that a combination of estrogen and progestin slightly increased the risk of heart attacks, so this treatment is not recommended.

Quit smoking. In smokers, HDL cholesterol levels average 4 mg/dL lower in men and 6 mg/dL lower in

This noninvasive, painless exam is carried out with a transducer, an instrument that transmits ultrasonic waves and receives the reflected echoes, which are recorded for analysis. The transducer is placed on various areas of the chest to create an image of the heart that is transmitted to a screen. If the doctor suspects valve dysfunction, endocarditis (infection of a heart valve), or a blood clot in one of the heart's chambers, and the echocardiogram does not provide sufficient information, a transducer can be introduced into the esophagus (the tube that connects the mouth to the stomach) to obtain a clearer image. This procedure is called transesophageal echocardiography, and it requires mild sedation.

Stress Echocardiography

In stress echocardiography, ultrasonic waves are used to image the heart at rest and then immediately following exercise. The technique can detect abnormalities in the motion of the heart wall. Abnormal motion at rest and during exercise indicates heart damage women than in nonsmokers, and quitting smoking tends to raise HDL cholesterol levels. Regular exposure to secondhand smoke also lowers HDL cholesterol. Using nicotine replacement therapy as an aid to stop smoking has no adverse effect on HDL cholesterol.

Exercise. Exercise can increase HDL cholesterol levels, but it must be performed regularly and at least at moderate intensity to significantly increase HDL cholesterol. One study showed that women who walked seven miles a week during a two-year period had no HDL increase, but another study revealed that those who ran seven miles per week had significant improvements in HDL.

Lose weight and make dietary changes. A higher body mass index is generally associated with lower HDL cholesterol levels, and studies show that weight loss may increase HDL cholesterol. However, weight loss achieved through diet alone appears not to improve HDL cholesterol as much as a combination of calorie restriction and physical activity.

Certain dietary changes may also be helpful. Avoid trans fatty acids, produced by hydrogenation of vegetable oils, which can lower HDL cholesterol levels. Trans fatty acids are found in margarines, and they are often used in baked products like cakes and cookies to extend their shelf life.

Although a reduction in the intake of saturated fat (found in animal and dairy products) and cholesterol lowers total and LDL cholesterol levels, these dietary measures can decrease HDL cholesterol as well, especially if saturated fats are replaced with carbohydrates. Instead, substitute some monounsaturated fat—found in foods such as olive and canola oils, almonds, and avocados—for saturated fat to maintain HDL levels.

Use alcohol moderately. A number of studies have found that moderate alcohol use raises HDL cholesterol, and population studies show that HDL cholesterol levels average 12% higher in people who drink moderately (about one or two drinks per day) than in those who abstain. According to one study, men who had at least two drinks a day had HDL cholesterol levels of 46 mg/dL, while nondrinkers had levels around 38 mg/dL. In addition, research clearly has shown that moderate alcohol intake is associated with a lower incidence of CHD. And the benefits appear to occur with all types of alcohol—not just red wine, as some reports have suggested.

However, because the risks associated with alcohol intake rise with increasing consumption, experts recommend that men drink no more than two drinks per day and women no more than one daily. Also, people with certain health conditions (such as liver disease or uncontrolled high blood pressure) or a personal or family history of alcoholism should not drink alcohol. Talk with your doctor about your level of alcohol consumption to be sure that, if you drink, you are not doing yourself more harm than good.

due to a prior heart attack. Normal motion at rest but abnormal motion during exercise indicates myocardial ischemia.

In stress echocardiography, people walk on a treadmill or pedal a stationary bicycle to raise their heart rate. When people are unable to raise their heart rate adequately through exercise, pharmacological stress echocardiography is performed. This procedure involves the administration of a drug such as dobutamine to raise the heart rate. If dobutamine does not adequately raise the heart rate, the drug atropine can be added. Alternatively, the drugs dipyridamole or adenosine can be used to raise the heart rate.

For many individuals, stress echocardiography is as accurate as a nuclear medicine stress test for detecting CHD. As with standard exercise stress testing using an ECG, there is a very small risk of a heart attack or cardiac arrest. Atropine can cause temporary dryness of the mouth, nose, throat, and skin. Dipyridamole and adenosine can cause flushing, chest pain, headache, shortness of breath, and loss of consciousness. For the side effects of dobutamine, see page 23.

Coronary Angiography

Coronary angiography is the "gold standard" method for assessing the extent of blockages in the coronary arteries. It is most often performed when an exercise or nuclear medicine stress test is abnormal, in order to identify the affected arteries and determine whether bypass surgery or angioplasty (see pages 51–58) is necessary. If angioplasty is required, it is often performed immediately after angiography.

During angiography, the doctor inserts a catheter into an artery in the groin and threads it up and into one of the coronary arteries (guided by images projected on a television screen). Injection of contrast material allows the detection of abnormalities in the coronary arteries on x-ray film.

The procedure lasts one to two hours and is usually performed in a cardiac catheterization laboratory in a hospital. Patients must remain in bed for six to eight hours afterward, with pressure maintained on the site where the catheter was inserted in the groin to prevent bleeding. Some patients require overnight hospitalization, but most can return home on the same day.

Angiography is associated with a small risk of allergic reactions or kidney failure (due to the injected contrast material) and infection or bleeding (due to damage to the arteries from the catheter). The risk of a heart attack or death from the procedure is about 1 in 1,000 when performed in a stable patient in a non-emergency situation.

Intravascular Ultrasound

Like angiography, intravascular ultrasound (IVUS) involves inserting a catheter into a coronary artery. But instead of using contrast material, sound waves create an image of the artery wall that allows the doctor to determine the amount of atherosclerotic plaque within the wall as well as the plaque's shape and composition. The procedure takes about 15 minutes.

IVUS is still an experimental procedure, but it appears to be safe and provides a more accurate picture of atherosclerosis in the coronary arteries than coronary angiography alone. The American College of Cardiology and the American Heart Association predict a continued increase in the use of IVUS for the diagnosis and treatment of CHD.

Electron-Beam Computed Tomography

Electron-beam computed tomography (EBCT), also known as ultrafast CT, is a noninvasive, 10- to 15-minute test that uses x-rays to

NEW RESEARCH

MRI Can Help Detect CHD

Using magnetic resonance imaging (MRI) to determine blood flow to the heart can help diagnose CHD by detecting blockages in the coronary arteries, research from Germany shows.

Advances in technology may soon allow doctors to use MRI to screen people suspected of having CHD, the investigators write. If MRI does not show decreased blood flow, the patient may not need to undergo more invasive tests like coronary angiography to diagnose CHD.

The research involved 84 people, average age 63, who were referred for diagnostic coronary angiography for suspected CHD. Before undergoing angiography, patients had an MRI to determine cardiac blood flow. The MRI was performed both while the patients were at rest and after they received a drug to mimic the effects of exercise on the heart.

The MRI predicted the presence of CHD in 89% of the 43 participants who had CHD detected by coronary angiography. The more arteries that were blocked, the more accurate the MRI.

The study authors conclude that, in some patients, MRI can detect blockages in the coronary arteries with a "a high diagnostic accuracy."

CIRCULATION
Volume 108, page 432
July 29, 2003

measure the amount of calcium in the coronary arteries. Calcium is a component of many (but not all) atherosclerotic plaques and is not present in healthy arteries.

Although EBCT can identify the presence of atherosclerotic plaque in the coronary arteries, it is unknown whether the test is any better at predicting CHD events than standard tests, such as measurements of blood pressure and blood lipids. In addition, the test is associated with a high number of false-positives—that is, it may indicate the presence of calcium when narrowing of the coronary arteries is not significant.

The American College of Cardiology and the American Heart Association do not recommend the use of EBCT in people at low risk for CHD who do not have symptoms.

Blood Markers of a Heart Attack

Damaged heart muscle releases certain proteins into the blood. These proteins include creatine kinase, creatine kinase-MB, troponin, and myoglobin, Measuring levels of these proteins with a series of blood tests may help diagnose a heart attack, as well as provide information about the person's expected outcome.

However, not all people having a heart attack have elevated levels of these proteins, especially soon after the onset of a heart attack. Also, some people have elevated levels because of other medical conditions. Therefore, blood markers are used in conjunction with the results of an ECG to determine whether a heart attack is in process.

Electrophysiology Studies

Electrophysiology studies are used to assess arrhythmias. A catheter is inserted into a vein in the groin and threaded up and into the heart. The catheter contains electrodes to stimulate and record the heart's electrical activity. The electrodes can be used to send electrical signals to the heart that reproduce arrhythmias. Medications can then be administered intravenously or orally to determine which ones prevent or suppress the arrhythmias.

Electrophysiology testing is much more helpful than an ECG in assessing arrhythmias because it allows doctors to pinpoint the origin of an abnormal heart rhythm and characterize the abnormality. It is also useful in deciding whether someone might benefit from an implantable cardioverter-defibrillator (see page 71). Not everybody with an arrhythmia needs to undergo electrophysiology testing. Most often it is used in people who have survived a cardiac arrest due to ventricular fibrillation or have experienced serious

NEW RESEARCH

Coronary Artery Calcium Helps Predict Heart Attacks

The presence of calcium in the coronary arteries is a strong predictor of who will experience CHD events, researchers report.

Men who were 30 to 76 years old with detectable coronary artery calcium were almost 11 times more likely to have a heart attack, undergo a coronary revascularization procedure (like angioplasty or bypass surgery), or die of CHD over a three-year period than those who did not have such calcium deposits. In women, the presence of coronary artery calcium was linked to a nearly threefold increased risk of CHD events.

The study followed 8,855 adults who had no symptoms of CHD but chose to undergo electron-beam computed tomography to detect coronary artery calcium. Coronary artery calcium may help doctors better determine the risk of CHD events among those at low to intermediate risk by traditional risk factor assessment.

According to an accompanying editorial, routine screening of all adults with electron-beam computed tomography "probably cannot be justified." People at high risk for CHD events will not need it, since they already require aggressive therapy. Those with a low risk of CHD events will likely not benefit, either. For those with an uncertain risk, screening for coronary artery calcium helps clarify that risk.

CIRCULATION
Volume 107, pages 2528 and 2571
May 27, 2003

rhythm disturbances such as ventricular tachycardia.

Because one of the objectives of electrophysiology testing may be to induce abnormal heart rhythms, the procedure takes place under carefully controlled conditions in a cardiac catheterization laboratory. A cardiologist specializing in electrophysiology performs the test, and the nurses and technicians who assist in the procedure are highly trained. The laboratory is equipped to treat a cardiac arrest or other serious complication. When performed by experts, the risk of complications is very small.

LIFESTYLE MEASURES TO PREVENT AND TREAT CORONARY HEART DISEASE

Lifestyle measures can have a greater impact on CHD than practically any other disease. The same lifestyle measures that are used to prevent CHD are also effective in preventing future events in people who already have CHD.

CHD is a progressive disorder: Once it develops, it can be controlled but not cured. A heart-healthy lifestyle is necessary to control the condition, even for people who are taking medication or have undergone surgery. For example, lifestyle changes may reduce the amount of cholesterol- or blood pressure-lowering medication needed. In turn, taking a lower dose of these drugs will reduce the risk of side effects. In addition, a combination of lifestyle changes and medication is often more effective than either alone.

The most effective lifestyle measures for the prevention and treatment of CHD are quitting smoking, eating a healthy diet (limiting intake of fat and sodium and increasing consumption of fiber, fruits, and vegetables), and engaging in regular physical activity.

Cigarette Smoking

Smoking is a difficult habit to break because of the powerful physical and psychological addiction to nicotine. In fact, only 8% of people who try to quit on their own are successful. But by using a combination of counseling, nicotine replacement therapy, and the prescription medication bupropion (Zyban), the odds of quitting increase to 35%. For information on smoking-cessation products and tips on quitting, see the feature on pages 14–15.

Dietary Fat

The average American diet contains about 35% to 40% of calories from fat. Not all of this fat is bad—in fact, some types of fat such as monounsaturated fat and omega-3 fatty acids have a beneficial effect on blood lipids and may lower the risk of developing or dying of CHD. But the prevalent type of fat in the American diet is saturated fat, which is a major dietary factor in raising blood cholesterol levels. Saturated fat includes most animal fats and some oils, such as palm and coconut oils.

The simplest dietary measure to lower the risk of CHD and CHD events is to limit total fat intake to less than 35% of calories and saturated fat to less than 10% of calories. These dietary measures help reduce blood cholesterol levels—specifically LDL cholesterol—and may also help people maintain an ideal weight (fat contains more calories than protein or carbohydrates). Also recommended is a reduction in dietary cholesterol to less than 300 mg per day. If LDL cholesterol levels remain high despite these dietary changes, saturated fat should be further restricted to less than 7% of calories and cholesterol to less than 200 mg per day.

Lowering fat intake to 15% or less of calories is not recommended, however. According to the American Heart Association, short-term studies show that such diets do not reduce LDL cholesterol levels any more than a standard low-fat diet. In addition, very-low-fat diets lower HDL cholesterol and increase triglyceride levels by up to 70%. People who are very young, are very old, or have type 1 diabetes should avoid very-low-fat diets because they may also lead to malnutrition.

When fat is consumed, monounsaturated fat should be chosen whenever possible so that it comprises 10% to 15% of calories. Olive and canola oils, almonds, and avocados contain large amounts of monounsaturated fat. When substituted for saturated fat in the diet, monounsaturated fat can lower LDL cholesterol levels, reduce the likelihood of LDL oxidation, and stabilize or even raise HDL cholesterol levels.

Polyunsaturated fat—found in safflower, sunflower, and corn oils—also lowers LDL cholesterol. A type of polyunsaturated fat known as omega-3 fatty acids lowers triglyceride levels and reduces the risk of dying from CHD. Foods rich in omega-3 fatty acids include fatty fish, such as herring, sardines, salmon, and mackerel. Omega-3 fatty acids are also present in certain plants (soybeans, walnuts, flaxseeds, and canola) and their oils. The American Heart Association recommends that people without CHD eat fish at least twice a week in addition to plant products high in omega-3 fatty acids. For those who already have CHD, the organization recommends the consumption of 1,000 mg of omega-3 fatty acids daily

NEW RESEARCH

Vitamin E, Beta-Carotene Do Not Prevent Heart Disease Deaths

Taking vitamin E or beta-carotene supplements does not reduce the risk of dying of CHD, a new analysis of previous research shows.

The analysis combined data from seven vitamin E trials and eight beta-carotene trials that tested the effect of these vitamins on various conditions, including CHD, stroke, lung cancer, skin cancer, and eye diseases. In each trial, over 1,000 older participants, randomized to receive a vitamin supplement or a placebo, were followed for 1½ to 12 years.

Vitamin E supplementation did not change the overall rate of death or death from CHD or stroke compared with a placebo. Beta-carotene was associated with slightly more deaths from any cause compared with a placebo (7.4% vs. 7%) and slightly more deaths from CHD or stroke compared with a placebo (3.4% vs. 3.1%). This small increase in risk in the beta-carotene group, which was highly significant, was partly due to the large number of smokers in the beta-carotene trials; beta-carotene is known to increase health risks in people who smoke.

Vitamin E supplements should not be used to prevent CHD or CHD events, the authors conclude. They further argue that the use of supplements containing beta-carotene or vitamin A should be "actively discouraged."

THE LANCET
Volume 361, page 2017
June 14, 2003

from fatty fish, fish oil supplements, or a combination of both. Always check with a doctor before beginning to take a fish oil supplement. For more information on omega-3 fatty acids, see the feature on pages 32–33.

To be avoided are trans fatty acids, which are found in foods made with hydrogenated or partially hydrogenated oils, such as margarine and commercial baked goods. Trans fatty acids are formed by adding hydrogen atoms to unsaturated oils to make them more saturated and therefore solid at room temperature and more shelf-stable. Trans fatty acids may be even more harmful than saturated fat because trans fatty acids not only raise LDL cholesterol but also lower HDL cholesterol more than saturated fat. The Institute of Medicine, a branch of the National Academy of Sciences, recommends that trans fatty acid consumption be as low as possible.

Dietary Sodium and Potassium

Limiting dietary sodium and increasing intake of potassium-rich foods can help control high blood pressure and, in turn, lower the risk of CHD and its progression.

The typical daily intake of sodium in the United States is 3,000 to 5,000 mg, although the body needs only about 200 mg of sodium a day. Limiting sodium intake typically lowers systolic blood pressure by 2 to 8 mm Hg and appears to be most effective in older individuals with high blood pressure. Experts recommend that people consume no more than 2,400 mg of sodium daily.

Salt added to foods during cooking or at the table is an obvious source of sodium in the diet. However, sodium occurs naturally in many foods and is used extensively in food processing. Cold cuts, canned vegetables, canned soups, cheeses, and snack foods can all be concentrated sources of sodium. Check nutrition labels for the amount of sodium in foods and choose low- or no-salt versions of packaged or processed foods, whenever possible.

A number of studies show that a low potassium intake can raise blood pressure, while increased potassium intake can lower blood pressure. People with high blood pressure should increase their intake of fresh fruits and vegetables, which are high in potassium and have the added benefit of being low in sodium and rich in dietary fiber and antioxidants. Citrus fruits and bananas are particularly good sources of potassium. Potassium supplements are not recommended for blood pressure control (unless prescribed by a doctor) and may even be dangerous for some people with high blood pressure.

Dietary Fiber and Soy

Experts recommend that everyone consume at least 25 to 30 g of dietary fiber each day. Both soluble and insoluble fiber are important, but soluble fiber is especially effective in lowering blood cholesterol levels. Foods containing soluble fiber—such as oats, oat bran, barley, legumes, prunes, apples, carrots, and grapefruits—should be included in the diet each day.

It is best to consume fiber from foods, which contain a variety of nutrients, rather than from supplements. But for people who find it difficult to get enough fiber from their diet, regular use of products that contain soluble fiber from psyllium seeds—such as Metamucil—can lower cholesterol levels by 5% to 10%.

Just how soluble fiber reduces cholesterol levels is unclear. Researchers theorize that soluble fiber works in much the same way as bile acid sequestrants (a class of lipid-lowering drugs)—by reducing the intestinal reabsorption of bile acids, which are made in the liver from cholesterol and released from the gallbladder into the intestine after meals. Normally, bile acids are reabsorbed from the intestine and returned to the liver for reprocessing. Bile acid sequestrants bind bile acids in the intestine and remove them via the stool. As a result, the liver converts more cholesterol to bile acids and removes more LDL from the blood.

Soy products also may lower blood cholesterol levels. In a recent analysis of 38 studies in which soy protein replaced animal protein in people's diets, eating an average of 47 g (about 10 oz.) of soy protein per day lowered total cholesterol by about 9%, LDL cholesterol by 13%, and triglycerides by 11%. Whether soy products lower cholesterol levels simply by substituting unsaturated fat for saturated fat (38% of the calories in soybeans come from fat, mostly unsaturated) or via isoflavones is not known. Isoflavones are naturally occurring estrogen-like compounds that are found in soy foods such as tofu and soy milk; estrogen lowers LDL cholesterol and boosts HDL cholesterol levels.

Antioxidants

Numerous studies have shown that people who eat a diet rich in fruits and vegetables are at reduced risk of developing CHD. Some researchers attribute this benefit to antioxidants. Antioxidants, which are plentiful in fruits and vegetables, help the body neutralize free radicals. Free radicals are by-products of normal metabolism that oxidize LDL and make it more likely to form deposits in the arteries.

In studies that measured blood levels of antioxidants, high levels

NEW RESEARCH

New Diet Similar to Drugs for Cholesterol Lowering

A vegetarian diet high in sterols, soy, fiber, and almonds can lower LDL cholesterol as much as treatment with a low-dose statin medication, according to a new study.

Forty-six participants, average age 59, with high LDL cholesterol levels underwent one of three treatments for four weeks: 1) a vegetarian control diet emphasizing whole grains and low-fat dairy products; 2) the vegetarian diet plus 20 mg of lovastatin (Mevacor) daily; or 3) an investigational vegetarian diet emphasizing sterols, soy protein, soluble fiber, and almonds.

LDL cholesterol levels decreased significantly more in the investigational-diet and lovastatin groups (29% and 31%, respectively) than in the control group (8%). (Higher doses or more potent statins can lower LDL cholesterol by 50%.) Similarly, levels of C-reactive protein, a risk factor for CHD, decreased significantly less in the control group (10%) than in the investigational-diet and lovastatin groups (28% and 33%, respectively).

Cholesterol guidelines recommend consuming 25 g of soluble fiber each day and possibly including 2 g of plant sterols daily. Levels of intake for soy and nuts have not been established, but the American Heart Association recognizes that these foods have potential heart benefits.

JOURNAL OF THE AMERICAN MEDICAL ASSOCIATION
Volume 290, pages 502 and 531
July 23/30, 2003

Stopping Fatal Heart Attacks With Fish

Eating foods rich in omega-3 fatty acids may reduce the risk of dying from coronary heart disease.

A line of research cast in the late 1970s has spawned a wealth of knowledge about a beneficial type of fat: omega-3 fatty acids. Found in fish and some plant products, these fats have been shown to lower the risk of sudden death from heart attacks in people with CHD. They may also benefit people at risk for CHD.

What Are Omega-3 Fatty Acids?

The three major types of highly unsaturated omega-3 fatty acids are eicosapentaenoic acid (EPA), docosahexaenoic acid (DHA), and alpha-linolenic acid (ALA). The only sources of EPA and DHA are fish (particularly fatty fish) and fish oils. (For a list of fish high in EPA and DHA, see the inset box on the opposite page.) ALA is found in certain plant and plant products, such as canola, soybeans, walnuts, and flaxseed, as well as the oils of these plants. Evidence is mounting that EPA and DHA can protect the heart; the data for ALA are not as strong.

The Evidence

Research into the heart benefits of omega-3 fatty acids began in the 1970s and 1980s when studies suggested that people who ate copious amounts of fish—for example, Japanese living in fishing villages and Greenland Eskimos—tended to have lower rates of atherosclerosis and heart attacks than Americans. Researchers hypothesized that the omega-3 fatty acids in fish might be responsible for this benefit.

A number of randomized clinical trials have examined the heart benefits of omega-3 fatty acid consumption in people diagnosed with CHD. A meta-analysis of these trials published in the *American Journal of Medicine* in 2002 reported that, in 11 randomized trials containing 15,806 people, omega-3 fatty acid-enriched diets or supplements decreased the risk of fatal heart attacks and sudden death from cardiac arrest by 30% and overall deaths by 20% compared with control diets or a placebo. However, the risk of nonfatal heart attacks was not significantly reduced.

How Do Omega-3 Fatty Acids Work?

Many experts suspect that the main mechanism by which omega-3 fatty acids reduce the risk of sudden death from CHD is by decreasing the heart's susceptibility to dangerous arrhythmias (irregular heart rhythms). The heart can begin to beat irregularly when it is subjected to stress, for example when it is not getting enough oxygen. These irregular heartbeats may lead to fatal ventricular fibrillation. Omega-3 fatty acids are incorporated into the membranes of cells in the heart, where they may stabilize the heart's rhythm.

Omega-3 fatty acids appear to have other beneficial effects on the heart. There is good evidence that they help reduce blood triglyceride levels. There is also some evidence, albeit less certain, that omega-3 fatty acids reduce the risk of blood clots, the growth of plaque in the arteries, high blood pressure, and inflammation, all of which contribute to atherosclerosis. They also appear to improve the function of blood vessels.

Getting Enough Omega-3 Fatty Acids

The average person in North America eats fish about once every 10 days and consumes about 1,600 mg of omega-3 fatty acids daily (about 200 mg of EPA and DHA combined and 1,400 mg of ALA). By contrast, the American Heart Association recommends that people not diagnosed with CHD eat fish, particularly those high in omega-3 fatty acids, at least twice weekly in addition to oils, nuts, and seeds high in ALA. For people who already have CHD, the organization recommends about 1,000 mg of EPA plus DHA per day from fatty fish, fish oil supplements, or a combination of both.

of vitamin C, vitamin E, and beta-carotene were associated with a reduced risk of CHD. Researchers hoped that supplements of these nutrients would slow the development of atherosclerosis in the coronary arteries by preventing LDL oxidation. However, three large trials have shown that vitamin E supplements provide no benefits in people with known CHD, and no studies have shown beneficial heart effects for supplemental vitamin C or beta-carotene.

Consequently, people should eat a diet rich in fruits and vegetables instead of relying on supplements to reduce their risk of CHD.

How the fish you eat is prepared may determine how well it protects against fatal CHD. In a study published in *Circulation* in March 2003, researchers found that people who ate broiled or baked fish three or more times per week had a 49% lower risk of fatal CHD and a 58% lower risk of death from a CHD-related arrhythmia than people who ate fish less than once a month. But people who ate fried fish or fish sandwiches experienced no reduced rate of CHD. Blood levels of omega-3 fatty acids were significantly higher in the people who consistently ate broiled or baked fish than in those who ate fried fish or fish sandwiches regularly. The researchers suggest that frying may reduce the omega-3 fatty acid content of fish. Another possible explanation is that the type of fish typically fried or used in fish sandwiches is not rich in omega-3 fatty acids.

Although current recommendations are that omega-3 fatty acids should preferably be obtained through food, some people may prefer fish oil supplements instead of, or in addition to, fish. Always consult your physician before beginning to take a fish oil supplement. Also, check the label of the supplement to determine its EPA and DHA content. A 1,000-mg fish oil capsule usually contains about 180 mg of EPA and 120 mg of DHA. This means that a person may have to take two to three capsules daily, in addition to eating fish regularly, to meet the American Heart Association's recommendation for omega-3 fatty acid intake for people with CHD.

Unfortunately, because the U.S. Food and Drug Administration does not regulate these supplements, different batches of the same brand may not contain the same levels of active ingredient. In addition, the content of EPA and DHA may not match the amount indicated on the label.

Potential Side Effects

One of the main concerns associated with eating large quantities of fish is that some species contain high levels of pollutants like methylmercury and polychlorinated biphenyls (PCBs). One recent study suggested that methylmercury exposure may increase the risk of CHD, while another found that methylmercury did not increase the risk.

Given the current data, experts say that the potential benefits of eating fish outweigh the possible risks for middle-aged and older men and for postmenopausal women. If you are concerned about exposure to pollutants, try to eat a variety of fish and avoid species like shark, swordfish, king mackerel, and tilefish. Fresh tuna is also high in methylmercury, and large amounts should probably be avoided; but canned tuna appears to be relatively safe.

Fish oil supplements are mercury free, but they can cause side effects such as nausea, gastrointestinal upset, and a fishy aftertaste. High intakes of omega-3 fatty acids from fish oil supplements (more than 3,000 mg per day of EPA plus DHA) are associated with an increased risk of bleeding and should be taken only under a doctor's supervision.

Good Sources of Omega-3 Fatty Acids (EPA and DHA)

Type of fish	EPA + DHA per 3 oz. serving
Herring	1,760 mg
Sardines	1,340 mg
Salmon	1,105 mg
Mackerel	955 mg
Trout	910 mg
Halibut	700 mg
Oysters	670 mg
Tuna	585 mg
Flounder	420 mg
King crab	350 mg
Shrimp	270 mg
Clams	240 mg
Lobster	240 mg
Haddock	200 mg
Cod	185 mg
Catfish	180 mg
Scallops	170 mg

Source: United States Department of Agriculture.

The U.S. Preventive Services Task Force concluded in July 2003 that there is insufficient evidence to recommend for or against vitamin C or E supplements for CHD prevention, and that beta-carotene supplements should be avoided because they can increase the risk of lung cancer in smokers.

Physical Activity

Regular exercise has many advantages. It helps to control body weight, can raise HDL cholesterol, improves the work capacity of the heart, reduces blood pressure, and relieves stress.

Many people believe that they must engage in strenuous physical activity for exercise to have any benefit. But even brisk walking can be a healthy form of exercise if performed regularly. One study of postmenopausal women found that physical activity equivalent to walking 30 to 45 minutes a day, three times a week, reduced the risk of a heart attack by 50%.

In 1995, the Centers for Disease Control and Prevention and the American College of Sports Medicine developed exercise recommendations. In reviewing all of the available evidence on physical activity and health, an expert panel convened by these two organizations concluded that adults should get 30 minutes or more of physical activity on most, preferably all, days of the week. The activity should be performed at moderate intensity—the equivalent of walking at a pace of three to four miles per hour.

In addition, the panel concluded that the 30 minutes of activity need not take place at one time. Short bursts of activity for 8 to 10 minutes, three times a day, are enough to reduce the risk of CHD, as long as they are performed at moderate intensity. Such activities include walking up stairs, walking short distances instead of driving, and doing calisthenics or pedaling a stationary bicycle while watching television. Gardening, housework, raking leaves, dancing, and playing with children can also count as part of the 30-minute total—if they are performed at a level of intensity that corresponds to brisk walking. Lower-intensity activities should be performed more often, for longer periods of time, or both.

The Institute of Medicine recently recommended getting even more exercise—an hour a day—but this goal is not realistic for most older Americans.

Men over age 40 and women over age 50 who plan to begin a vigorous exercise program should consult their doctor first, particularly if they have been leading a sedentary lifestyle. Those who have CHD or are at high risk for developing it should also see a doctor before beginning any new physical activities, even moderate ones. Though rare, heart attacks may be triggered by unusually high amounts of exertion in people with an otherwise sedentary lifestyle. Thus, physical activity should be incorporated gradually into one's lifestyle, and intensity increased slowly and steadily.

Weight Control

A low-fat diet combined with regular exercise will help people maintain an appropriate weight or lose weight, if necessary. Weight

NEW RESEARCH

Leisure-Time Exercise Most Beneficial

Even moderate leisure-time exercise can reduce the risk of CHD, but physically demanding jobs provide no such benefits and may even increase the risk, according to a German study. Although the findings reinforce widely held beliefs about the association between fitness and well-being, the connection between workplace exertion and CHD risk was somewhat surprising, the study's authors say.

More than 300 people with stable CHD were compared with 479 healthy individuals; both groups were interviewed about their physical activity at work and at play. People who exercised for two or more hours weekly during their free time were 61% to 73% less likely to have CHD than those who never exercised. Getting a lesser amount of exercise also decreased the risk of CHD but not as dramatically. Interestingly, participants who reported any amount of physical exertion on the job were more likely to have CHD.

The results, note the authors, demonstrate that even simple activities, such as low-intensity walking or bike riding, can have a profoundly positive impact on health. They also hypothesize that differences between the nature of work-related and leisure-time activities may be responsible for the different effects they had on CHD risk.

ARCHIVES OF INTERNAL MEDICINE
Volume 163, page 1200
May 26, 2003

loss is the most effective way to lower elevated triglyceride levels. It also helps to raise HDL cholesterol: In one study, a 5-lb. weight gain lowered HDL levels by 4% in men and 2% in women; losing weight counteracted this effect.

Weight loss is one of the first steps in the treatment of type 2 diabetes, and a weight loss of as little as 5 to 10 lbs. may lower blood pressure enough to make blood pressure-lowering medications unnecessary. Blood pressure drops even more with a combination of weight loss and medication than with medication alone.

Alcohol

Moderate alcohol consumption is associated with a decreased risk of CHD, possibly because alcohol increases HDL cholesterol levels, inhibits the constriction of coronary arteries, and limits blood clot formation. But because of the health risks of alcohol—heavy drinking can damage the heart and liver and cause accidents and hemorrhagic (bleeding) strokes—the American Heart Association does not recommend drinking alcohol to reduce the risk of CHD. In fact, controlling other risk factors for CHD, such as quitting smoking, improving blood lipids, and lowering blood pressure, has a greater impact on CHD risk than moderate alcohol consumption.

The American Heart Association says that people who drink infrequently should not begin to drink more regularly to reduce their risk of CHD. Men who drink regularly should consume no more than two drinks a day (one drink equals 12 oz. of beer, 5 oz. of wine, or 1½ oz. of 80-proof spirits); women should limit their intake to one a day. And some people should avoid alcohol altogether. These include people with elevated blood triglyceride levels or uncontrolled high blood pressure; those with liver disease, heart failure, or a family or personal history of alcohol abuse; and pregnant women.

Stress Reduction

People can cope with stress in a variety of ways. Regular aerobic exercise—even a daily walk after work—can ease stress. A support network of family and friends can also help reduce stress. Relaxation techniques such as yoga, tai chi, and transcendental meditation, as well as more formal programs in which relaxation exercises are taught by a therapist, can be useful as well. Some people may benefit from behavior modification techniques—for example, biofeedback, anxiety management, and stress management.

NEW RESEARCH

Increasing Physical Activity Can Add Years to Life

An increase in the amount of exercise performed each day—even small increases in walking—may lengthen the life span of older women who are sedentary.

Physical activity was assessed initially and after six years in a study of 9,518 women, age 65 and older. Sedentary women who increased the distance they walked daily by one mile during the follow-up had 48% fewer deaths from any cause, 36% fewer deaths from heart attack and stroke, and 51% fewer deaths from cancer compared with women who remained sedentary. And the more the women increased their physical activity, the greater their reduction in cardiovascular mortality during the 12½-year study.

The decreased risk of death linked to increases in physical activity could have resulted from numerous factors, such as a reduction in risk factors for heart attack and stroke, better fitness of the heart and lungs, and fewer falls (and therefore fewer fractures and less physical disability).

Because active women who became sedentary during the study had death rates similar to women who were sedentary throughout the study, current physical activity, rather than a history of being active, is important in determining the occurrence of events that may shorten life span.

JOURNAL OF THE AMERICAN MEDICAL ASSOCIATION
Volume 289, page 2379
May 14, 2003

Homocysteine

Homocysteine levels can be lowered with folic acid supplements, but to date no proof exists that this therapy will reduce the risk of CHD. People concerned about their homocysteine levels can safely take 400 to 800 micrograms of folic acid daily, either as a single tablet or in a multivitamin. Folic acid should be taken along with 1 mg of vitamin B_{12} since it can mask the typical blood changes of pernicious anemia, which is caused by a lack of vitamin B_{12}. Taking 50 mg a day of vitamin B_6 is often recommended as well.

THE BENEFITS OF LOWERING CHOLESTEROL LEVELS

The benefits of improving lipid levels with diet and medication have been clearly demonstrated by a number of well-designed studies. The results depend on whether or not someone has been diagnosed with CHD and whether CHD risk factors are present.

No known CHD. Improving lipid levels has been shown to benefit people with no history of CHD. In one trial from Oslo, men were able to reduce their total cholesterol levels by 10% and their risk of death by 47% over five years using diet alone. Results with medication also have been dramatic. One drug trial found that CHD events decreased by 2% for every 1% drop in total cholesterol. In a study of Scottish men, medication reduced overall mortality by 22% over a five-year period. More recently, in the Air Force/Texas Coronary Atherosclerosis Prevention Study, men and women with low HDL cholesterol levels who took lovastatin (Mevacor) for five years had a 40% reduction in heart attacks compared with those who received a placebo. And in the Helsinki Heart Study, men with elevated triglyceride levels who took gemfibrozil (Lopid) had a 34% reduction in nonfatal heart attacks and CHD-related deaths after five years compared with the placebo group.

Known CHD. Studies show that cholesterol-lowering drugs called statins slow the progression of atherosclerotic plaques, promote plaque regression, and prevent the formation of new plaques in both men and women with CHD. These improvements can occur within two years of beginning treatment.

Four large trials, each lasting at least five years, have demonstrated the benefits of lowering LDL cholesterol levels with statins in people with CHD. In the Scandinavian Simvastatin Survival Study (4S), the risk of a heart attack was reduced by 27%, the risk of dying of a heart attack was lowered by 42%, and the need for angioplasty or bypass surgery was decreased by 37% in people taking simvastatin (Zocor), compared with those taking a placebo. Lowering cholesterol levels also reduced deaths from all causes by 30% in men. The overall death rate was not lowered in the women, however, possibly because there were too few CHD deaths to see an effect.

Participants in the Cholesterol and Recurrent Events (CARE) study also had CHD, but their starting levels of cholesterol were lower than those of the participants in the 4S trial. Nonetheless, the incidence of CHD events and the need for angioplasty or bypass surgery was lower in the pravastatin (Pravachol) group than in the placebo group over a five-year period, and women benefited more than men. The overall death rate, however, was not reduced in this study.

In the Long Term Intervention with Pravastatin in Ischemic Disease (LIPID) trial, which looked at people with CHD and cholesterol levels between 155 and 271 mg/dL, pravastatin lowered the number of CHD events, the need for angioplasty or bypass surgery, and overall mortality over a six-year period.

The Heart Protection Study, the largest and most recent trial to evaluate the benefits of statins in people with CHD, found that simvastatin reduced the risk of a heart attack, angioplasty, or bypass surgery by 25% and the risk of CHD-related death by 18% over a five-year period, compared with a placebo. Simvastatin helped prevent CHD events in men and women of all ages—even in those with desirable LDL cholesterol levels (less than 100 mg/dL).

The incidence of ischemic strokes (strokes caused by a clot in an artery carrying blood to the brain) also fell significantly in those taking a statin in all four trials.

Another type of cholesterol-lowering drug called gemfibrozil also is beneficial for people with CHD. In one study of more than 2,500 men with elevated triglyceride levels, those who took gemfibrozil for five years had a 24% reduction in nonfatal heart attacks and CHD-related deaths, compared with those who took a placebo. Further analysis of the data revealed that the reduction in CHD events with gemfibrozil was due to an increase in HDL cholesterol levels and that men with diabetes or insulin resistance benefited the most from the drug.

MEDICATIONS TO PREVENT OR TREAT CORONARY HEART DISEASE

Lifestyle changes may be all that are needed to control blood lipid levels and high blood pressure, but when they fail to do so, medication can be used in addition to lifestyle changes. Drugs may also be needed to relieve angina and to reduce the ability of the blood to form clots.

Lipid-Lowering Medications

If three to six months of a low-fat, low-cholesterol diet fail to adequately lower blood cholesterol levels, drugs may be prescribed in addition to lifestyle changes. Five classes of lipid-lowering drugs are available: HMG-CoA reductase inhibitors, better known as statins; bile acid sequestrants; nicotinic acid, or niacin; fibrates; and cholesterol absorption inhibitors. (See the chart on pages 42–43.)

Although cholesterol-lowering medications are frequently prescribed to people with elevated cholesterol levels, they are greatly underprescribed after a heart attack. No more than 30% to 50% of heart attack patients who should be on lipid-lowering therapy currently receive these drugs. Moreover, studies have shown that as many as half of people discontinue lipid-lowering medications after one year, even though these drugs should be taken indefinitely.

HMG-CoA reductase inhibitors (statins). Statins are the most effective drugs for lowering total and LDL cholesterol. They produce about a 30% to 50% reduction in LDL cholesterol levels, a 5% to 10% increase in HDL cholesterol levels, and a 10% to 25% reduction in triglyceride levels. The statins include atorvastatin (Lipitor), fluvastatin (Lescol), lovastatin (Mevacor), pravastatin (Pravachol), simvastatin (Zocor), and the newly approved rosuvastatin (Crestor). Cerivastatin (Baycol) was taken off the market in 2001 after it was linked to fatal kidney disease due to severe muscle inflammation. Lovastatin is the only statin available as a generic. A combination of lovastatin and extended-release niacin (Advicor) is also available.

In addition to their positive effects on blood lipid levels, statins appear to improve the function of the endothelium in the arteries. Specifically, they help arteries regain at least some of their normal ability to widen and permit increased blood flow during exercise. Statins also reduce the risk of plaque rupture by decreasing inflammation within the walls of arteries.

Side effects are uncommon, occurring in only 1% to 2% of people. The most common side effect is muscle aches. Others include bloating or gas, heartburn, nausea, allergic reactions, stomach pain, and increases in liver enzymes. In rare cases, the kidneys can become damaged by severe muscle inflammation. Call your doctor if you experience fever and unusual or unexplained muscle aches while taking a statin.

How Statins Help Control Blood Cholesterol Levels

Statin medications are among the most widely prescribed drugs in the world. Here's how they work.

Cholesterol is an essential component of cell membranes. It is also required to form hormones and bile acids; the latter help the body to absorb dietary fats from the intestine. But too much cholesterol in the blood can lead to a buildup of atherosclerotic plaques within the walls of arteries. These plaques are potentially dangerous; they can impede blood flow to the heart, brain, and other organs, or they can rupture and lead to a blood clot that may cause a heart attack or stroke.

Statins (also called HMG-CoA reductase inhibitors) are drugs that decrease blood levels of total cholesterol and low density lipoprotein (LDL, or "bad") cholesterol. They may also reduce triglyceride levels and raise high density lipoprotein (HDL, or "good") cholesterol levels. Depending on the dose, statins can reduce LDL cholesterol and triglycerides by as much as 50% and 25%, respectively, and may increase HDL cholesterol by 10%. The ways that statins alter cholesterol levels and prevent cardiovascular disease are as follows.

The liver makes 80% of the cholesterol in the body. The remainder comes from cholesterol in the diet. Statins work in the liver by blocking HMG-CoA reductase, an enzyme that controls the rate of cholesterol production. By binding to this enzyme, statins prevent it from converting HMG-CoA to mevalonate.

Because mevalonate is required for the synthesis of cholesterol, statins reduce the liver's production of cholesterol. But the liver still needs cholesterol, so it generates extra receptors to grab LDL cholesterol from the blood as it flows by. Statins also raise blood levels of HDL, which carries cholesterol from the body's tissues and from atherosclerotic plaques to the liver. As a result of the fall in LDL cholesterol and increase in HDL, plaque formation in the arteries is slowed and the cholesterol component of plaque may be decreased.

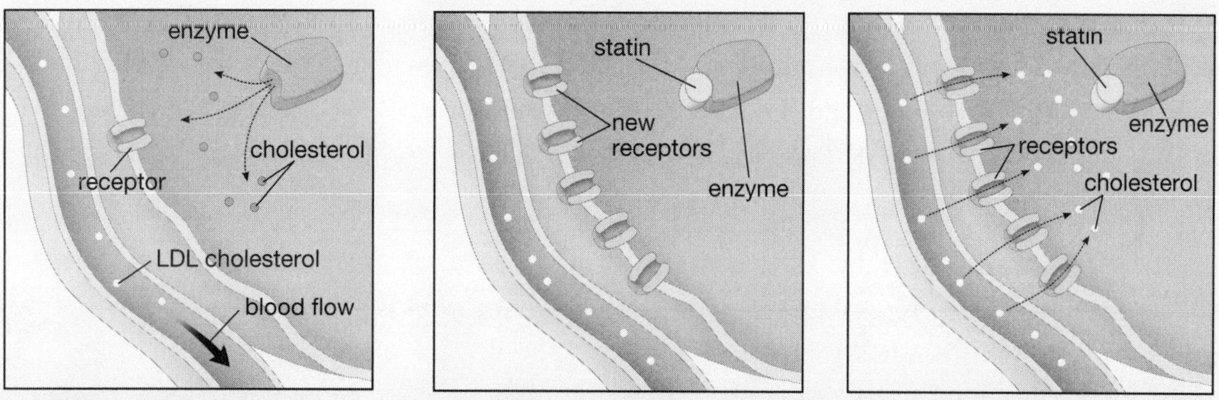

An enzyme called HMG-CoA reductase in the liver controls the body's rate of cholesterol production.

Statins bind to the enzyme and reduce the production of cholesterol. New receptors form to supply the liver with cholesterol from the bloodstream.

LDL cholesterol moves from the bloodstream through the receptors and into the liver, lowering the amount of LDL in the blood.

Bile acid sequestrants. The bile acid sequestrants, cholestyramine (Questran) and colestipol (Colestid), have proven long-term safety and effectiveness. A newer bile acid sequestrant called colesevelam (WelChol) became available in 2000. Combinations of bile acid sequestrants with statins or nicotinic acid are especially effective in lowering LDL cholesterol levels. Such combinations have been shown in a number of studies to slow the progression—or even cause regression—of plaques. Bile acid sequestrants can cause triglyceride levels to rise, however.

Common side effects include constipation, heartburn, bloating, belching, abdominal discomfort, and irritation of the anal area. Intestinal obstruction is a rare adverse effect; stop taking the bile acid sequestrant and contact your doctor if you experience severe abdominal pain. Rarely, bile acid sequestrants can interfere with the absorption of folic acid. Taking bile acid sequestrants at the proper times is important to avoid interference with the absorption of other drugs.

Nicotinic acid (niacin). Large doses of this B vitamin are the most effective therapy to raise HDL cholesterol. The drug also can lower triglycerides and LDL cholesterol.

Nicotinic acid frequently causes adverse effects. Skin flushing and itching are common but not dangerous. More serious side effects include liver toxicity, peptic ulcers (ulcers in the stomach or upper intestine), gout, and an increase in blood glucose levels. Nicotinic acid should not be taken by those with current or past peptic ulcers, liver disease, or gout. It should be used with caution in people with diabetes or pre-diabetes.

Extended-release niacin (Niaspan) is associated with less flushing than immediate-release niacin (Niacor) and has the added advantage of once-a-day dosing at bedtime, rather than three times a day with meals. Older, sustained-release niacin preparations increase the risk of liver toxicity and should be avoided. Although niacin is available over the counter, all preparations should be used under a doctor's supervision.

Fibrates. The fibrates, fenofibrate (Lofibra, Tricor) and gemfibrozil (Lopid), are the treatment of choice for people with markedly increased blood triglyceride levels. But any reduction in triglycerides with fibrates may be accompanied by a rise in total and LDL cholesterol levels. When this problem occurs, the addition of a statin can improve LDL cholesterol levels but may cause muscle inflammation in about 1% of people. Muscle inflammation is reversible, but both drugs must be promptly discontinued, since persistent, severe muscle inflammation can cause kidney failure. Call your doctor right away if you experience a fever and unusual or unexplained muscle aches. Other possible side effects of fibrates include diarrhea, nausea, gas, skin rash, infection, and flu-like symptoms.

Cholesterol absorption inhibitors. Cholesterol absorption inhibitors are the newest class of lipid-lowering drugs. As their name implies, these drugs work by blocking the absorption of dietary

NEW RESEARCH

New Statin More Effective Than Others for Lowering LDL Cholesterol

Rosuvastatin (Crestor)—a new statin approved by the FDA in 2003—may be more effective at low doses than other statins for lowering LDL cholesterol and raising HDL cholesterol.

In a study of 2,431 people with high LDL cholesterol levels (160 to 250 mg/dL), researchers compared the effects of 10 to 40 mg of rosuvastatin daily with those of 10 to 80 mg of atorvastatin (Lipitor), 10 to 80 mg of simvastatin (Zocor), and 10 to 40 mg of pravastatin (Pravachol).

After six weeks, at equivalent doses rosuvastatin lowered LDL cholesterol 8% more than atorvastatin, up to 18% more than simvastatin, and 26% more than pravastatin. HDL cholesterol rose significantly more with rosuvastatin (8% to 10%) than with the other drugs (2% to 7%).

Unlike other statins, however, no clinical trials have been completed that show the effect of rosuvastatin on CHD. Similarly, the safety of rosuvastatin hasn't been fully established, whereas the safety of the other statins—which have been taken by millions of people for many years—is clear.

Side effects of rosuvastatin are uncommon and similar to those of other statins. The greatest risk is muscle inflammation, which can occur with all the statins, especially when taken with fibrates, antifungal drugs, or cyclosporine.

THE AMERICAN JOURNAL OF CARDIOLOGY
Volume 92, page 152
July 15, 2003

cholesterol from the small intestine. Ezetimibe (Zetia) is the first drug to be approved in this class. Studies show that ezetimibe lowers total cholesterol, LDL cholesterol, and triglycerides when used alone or in combination with a statin. Side effects of ezetimibe are infrequent and include back pain, joint pain, diarrhea, and sinus inflammation.

Cholesterol-lowering margarines. In 1999, the U.S. Food and Drug Administration (FDA) approved cholesterol-lowering food additives called stanols and sterols, which are used in the margarines Benecol and Take Control. These margarines can reduce LDL cholesterol by 7% to 14% when used daily in combination with a low-fat, low-cholesterol diet and regular exercise for a year or longer. The margarines cost around $5 for a week's supply.

Antihypertensive Medications

The following five classes of drugs, used individually or in combination, are most frequently prescribed for the treatment of high blood pressure: diuretics, beta-blockers, ACE inhibitors, angiotensin II receptor blockers, and calcium channel blockers.

Diuretics. By increasing the amount of sodium excreted in the urine, diuretics promote water loss and decrease blood volume. Diuretics can also widen small blood vessels, which increases blood flow. Thiazides are the most commonly used diuretics. They have the advantages of low cost and once-a-day dosing.

Possible side effects include weakness; fatigue; erectile dysfunction; a rise in blood glucose, uric acid, and triglyceride levels; a lowering of HDL cholesterol levels; and excessive loss of potassium in the urine. Potassium depletion can be prevented by combining a thiazide diuretic with a potassium-sparing diuretic such as triamterene (Dyrenium) or by taking potassium supplements.

Thiazide diuretics are usually the first medication tried in people with high blood pressure. In addition to their blood pressure-lowering effect, these drugs may lower the risk of heart attacks, heart failure, and strokes. In a recent study called the Antihypertensive and Lipid-Lowering Treatment to Prevent Heart Attack Trial (ALLHAT), people taking a thiazide diuretic had the same risk of death and nonfatal heart attacks as people taking an ACE inhibitor or calcium channel blocker.

Beta-blockers. These drugs, which block the actions of epinephrine (adrenaline), lower blood pressure by slowing heart rate and decreasing cardiac output (the amount of blood pumped by the heart). Beta-blockers also can alleviate angina, help treat heart failure, and,

NEW RESEARCH

Statin Plus Ezetimibe Better Than Either Drug Alone To Lower LDL

Combining the statin atorvastatin (Lipitor) with the new cholesterol-lowering medication ezetimibe (Zetia) lowers LDL cholesterol levels better than taking either drug alone.

The effectiveness of two drugs together may be explained by the fact that they have different mechanisms of action: Atorvastatin blocks production of cholesterol by the liver, and ezetimibe blocks absorption of cholesterol from the intestine.

In a new study, researchers randomly assigned 628 adults with elevated LDL cholesterol levels to take a placebo, atorvastatin alone, ezetimibe alone, or a combination of atorvastatin and ezetimibe.

After 12 weeks of treatment, people taking the combination treatment had a 55% reduction in LDL cholesterol levels, compared with a 42% reduction in the atorvastatin-alone group and an 18% reduction in the ezetimibe-alone group. The combination treatment also raised HDL cholesterol levels and lowered total cholesterol, triglyceride, and C-reactive protein levels significantly better than either agent alone.

The percentage of patients who experienced treatment-related side effects was similar in the atorvastatin group and the combination group (17% vs. 23%).

CIRCULATION
Volume 107, page 2409
May 20, 2003

Lipid-Lowering Drugs 2004

Drug Type	Generic Name	Brand Name	Average Daily Dosage*	Estimated Cost (Generic Cost)†
HMG-CoA reductase inhibitors (statins)	atorvastatin	Lipitor	10 to 80 mg	10 mg: $250
	fluvastatin	Lescol	20 to 80 mg	40 mg: $178
	fluvastatin, extended-release	Lescol XL	80 mg	80 mg: $228
	lovastatin§	Mevacor	20 to 80 mg	20 mg: $268 ($238)
	pravastatin	Pravachol	10 to 40 mg	40 mg: $452
	rosuvastatin	Crestor	5 to 40 mg	10 mg: $263
	simvastatin	Zocor	10 to 80 mg	20 mg: $458
Bile acid sequestrants	cholestyramine	Questran	8 to 24 g	4 g‡: $278 ($186)
		Questran Light	8 to 24 g	4 g‡: $280 ($186)
	colestipol	Colestid	10 to 30 g	5 g‡: $148
		Colestid Flavored	10 to 30 g	5 g‡: $177
		Colestid pills	10 to 30 g	1 g: $55
	colesevelam	WelChol	3.75 to 4.375 g	625 mg: $79
Nicotinic acid	niacin	Niacor	3 to 6 g	500 mg: $28 ($4)
	niacin, extended-release§	Niaspan	375 to 1,000 mg	500 mg: $99
Fibrates	fenofibrate	Lofibra	67 to 200 mg	67 mg: $82
		Tricor	54 to 160 mg	54 mg: $99
	gemfibrozil	Lopid	1200 mg	600 mg: $166 ($116)
Cholesterol absorption inhibitor	ezetimibe	Zetia	10 mg	10 mg: $241

* These dosages represent an average range for the treatment of elevated lipid levels. The precise effective dosage varies from patient to patient and depends on many factors. Do not make any changes in your medication without consulting your doctor.

† Average wholesale prices to pharmacists for 100 tablets or capsules (unless otherwise indicated) of the dosage strength listed. Costs to consumers are higher. If a generic version is available, the cost is listed in parentheses. Source: *Red Book, 2003* (Medical Economics Data, publishers).

‡ Refers to the amount of the active ingredient.

§ A combination of lovastatin and extended-release niacin (Advicor) is available.

How They Work	Advantages	Disadvantages
HMG-CoA reductase is required for the liver to produce cholesterol. Statins block the action of this enzyme. As a result, the liver makes less cholesterol and more LDL receptors, which remove LDL from the blood.	The most effective drugs to lower total and LDL cholesterol. Can lower LDL by 30% to 50% and triglycerides by 10% to 25%. Can increase HDL cholesterol by 5% to 10%. Side effects are uncommon. Better tolerated than bile acid sequestrants or nicotinic acid. Reduce the risk of heart attacks, strokes, and death.	Gastrointestinal symptoms or reversible liver injury occur in 1% to 2% of people. Muscle soreness also can occur, more often when statins are used in combination with nicotinic acid, fibrates, erythromycin, antifungal agents, or cyclosporine. When severe, muscle inflammation can cause kidney damage.
Bile acids, made from cholesterol by the liver, are released from the gallbladder into the intestine after meals. Normally, bile acids are reabsorbed from the intestine and returned to the liver for reprocessing. Bile acid sequestrants bind bile acids in the intestine and remove them via the stool. As a result, the liver converts more cholesterol to bile acids and removes more LDL from the blood.	Long-term safety and effectiveness have been established. Can be combined with any other lipid-lowering drug. Used for people with elevated LDL cholesterol levels but normal triglyceride levels. On average, bile acid sequestrants reduce LDL cholesterol by 15% to 25%. Used alone, these drugs reduce the risk of heart attacks. Bile acid sequestrants also slow the progression of plaques and may even cause plaque regression when combined with other cholesterol-lowering drugs.	Constipation is common, especially at higher doses. This side effect may be temporary and can be relieved with a high-fiber diet or stool-softening pills. May cause heartburn or a feeling of fullness. Triglyceride levels may rise. Rarely, bile acid sequestrants can interfere with the absorption of folic acid. Proper timing of drug dosage is important to avoid interference with the absorption of other drugs.
Nicotinic acid decreases the production of VLDL by the liver. VLDL is the major carrier of triglycerides in the blood.	Safe and effective, niacin is used to treat high LDL cholesterol levels, high triglyceride levels, and low HDL cholesterol levels. The most effective drug to raise HDL levels (about 20% on average), it also reduces LDL cholesterol on average by 10% to 20% and triglycerides by 20% to 30%. Used alone, it decreases heart attacks and heart attack deaths. When combined with bile acid sequestrants, it slows progression and contributes to regression of plaques in the coronary arteries.	Skin flushing and itching may occur about half an hour after taking the drug. These side effects often decrease with time and can be greatly reduced by starting on a low dose and gradually increasing the dose, taking an extended-release formulation, taking the drug with meals, or taking an aspirin half an hour before taking the drug. Should not be used by people with peptic ulcers or a history of ulcers or by people with gout. Should be used with caution in people with diabetes or pre-diabetes. In rare cases, sustained-release formulations can cause liver injury.
These drugs stimulate the activity of lipoprotein lipase. This enzyme breaks down triglycerides and thus lowers VLDL and triglyceride levels.	Fibrates are safe for long-term use. They are the most effective drugs to lower triglycerides, producing reductions of 30% to 50% or more. They also raise HDL cholesterol by about 10%. Fenofibrate may be more effective than gemfibrozil in lowering total and LDL cholesterol. Gemfibrozil reduces the risk of heart attacks.	In some people, total and LDL cholesterol levels may increase. Feelings of fullness, diarrhea, or gas may occur. May cause muscle aches. May cause reversible liver injury. Long-term use can lead to gallstones. Doses should be reduced in individuals with kidney dysfunction.
Ezetimibe inhibits the absorption of dietary cholesterol in the small intestine.	Safe and effective, ezetimibe lowers total cholesterol by 13%, LDL cholesterol by 18%, and triglycerides by 8%. Greater reductions in total cholesterol, LDL cholesterol, and triglycerides are achieved when used in combination with a statin. May be useful in people who experience intolerable side effects with statins or cannot reach desirable lipid levels with a statin alone.	People with liver disease or elevated liver enzymes should not take ezetimibe in combination with a statin. Side effects are uncommon; they include back pain, joint pain, diarrhea, and sinus inflammation.

in people who have had a heart attack, reduce the risk of death and future heart attacks.

Possible adverse effects of beta-blockers include fatigue, depression, erectile dysfunction, a rise in blood glucose and triglyceride levels, a fall in HDL cholesterol levels, and wheezing in people with bronchospastic diseases such as asthma. In people taking insulin or certain oral diabetes drugs, beta-blockers may mask the warning symptoms of hypoglycemia (low blood sugar).

ACE inhibitors. ACE stands for angiotensin-converting enzyme. One way ACE inhibitors decrease blood pressure is by inhibiting the formation of angiotensin II, a substance that constricts blood vessels and stimulates the adrenal glands to release aldosterone, a hormone that promotes sodium retention.

ACE inhibitors are also effective for the prevention of heart failure in people with impaired heart function (for example, those who have suffered a heart attack), as well as for the treatment of heart failure. The Health Outcomes Prevention Evaluation (HOPE) study showed that the ACE inhibitor ramipril (Altace) significantly reduced the risk of CHD events over a five-year period in people with known CHD or with diabetes plus one of the following CHD risk factors: high blood pressure, elevated total cholesterol levels, cigarette smoking, low HDL cholesterol levels, or microalbuminuria (protein in the urine). ACE inhibitors may also reduce the risk of diabetes, kidney disease, and strokes.

ACE inhibitors cause fewer adverse effects than diuretics or beta-blockers; a dry cough is the most frequent side effect. People who develop a cough may take an angiotensin II receptor blocker instead. Uncommon problems of ACE inhibitors are an increase in blood potassium levels and impaired kidney function. Women who are pregnant or planning on becoming pregnant should not take ACE inhibitors.

Angiotensin II receptor blockers. These drugs lower blood pressure by interfering with the action of angiotensin II. They may also halt the proliferation of smooth muscle cells in blood vessel walls.

Researchers are studying whether these drugs can also protect the heart. One recent study found that an angiotensin II receptor blocker was helpful in the treatment of heart failure. There is also some evidence that angiotensin II receptor blockers may help prevent diabetes, kidney disease in people with diabetes, and strokes in people at high risk.

Side effects include headache and digestive upset, although these problems occurred at about the same frequency in people taking a placebo in one study. Like ACE inhibitors, angiotensin II receptor blockers should not be used by pregnant women or women planning a pregnancy.

Calcium channel blockers. These drugs lower blood pressure by dilating arteries and, possibly, by decreasing cardiac output. These agents help alleviate the symptoms of angina. They are also sometimes used to reduce the risk of strokes and kidney disease.

Long-acting calcium channel blockers are used because they are safer and more effective than short-acting calcium channel blockers. Long-acting calcium channel blockers also need to be taken only once a day, reducing the likelihood of missed doses. Flushing and swelling of the legs are occasional side effects.

Antiplatelet and Anticoagulant Drugs

Antiplatelet and anticoagulant drugs reduce the formation of blood clots. Antiplatelet drugs, which work by preventing platelets from clumping together, include aspirin, clopidogrel (Plavix), abciximab (ReoPro), eptifibatide (Integrilin), and tirofiban (Aggrastat). Anticoagulant drugs such as warfarin (Coumadin) work by inhibiting the formation of fibrin, a protein involved in blood clotting.

Long-term aspirin therapy reduces the risk of heart attacks, strokes, and death. Aspirin is routinely prescribed to people who have had a heart attack. It is also recommended for some people who have no signs of CHD or other cardiovascular disease but have one or more risk factors for a heart attack. Men age 40 and older, postmenopausal women, smokers, and people with high blood pressure, diabetes, high total or LDL cholesterol levels, low HDL cholesterol levels, or a family history of heart attacks before age 55 in men and age 65 in women should talk to their doctor about taking aspirin to prevent a heart attack.

Aspirin is also used to reduce the risk of strokes in people with atrial fibrillation. In addition, chewing a regular-dose aspirin immediately after the onset of heart attack symptoms increases the chances of survival. One study found that people who chewed an aspirin at the time of a heart attack had a 25% lower risk of death from CHD than those who did not chew an aspirin.

Because aspirin can increase the risk of gastrointestinal bleeding and hemorrhagic stroke, individuals with a history of bleeding in the gastrointestinal tract, those with uncontrolled high blood pressure, and those who take nonsteroidal anti-inflammatory drugs (NSAIDs) or anticoagulant drugs should take aspirin with caution or not at all.

Clopidogrel is mainly used for two to four weeks after angioplasty with stent placement (see pages 54–58). A recent study demonstrated a benefit when clopidogrel was taken with aspirin for several months by people with unstable angina. Common side effects of clopidogrel include nausea, upset stomach, stomach pain, diarrhea, rash, and itchy skin.

Three new antiplatelet agents—abciximab, eptifibatide, and tirofiban—are administered intravenously in people undergoing angioplasty and in those with unstable angina. These drugs may cause excessive bleeding.

The anticoagulant warfarin is used in heart attack patients with evidence of a blood clot inside the heart and in those with markedly impaired heart function. Patients with atrial fibrillation also are treated with warfarin, especially if they have other risk factors for a stroke. The risk of excessive bleeding, the most common side effect of warfarin, can be reduced with periodic blood tests to measure how quickly the blood clots.

Hormone Replacement Therapy

Estrogen is effective in relieving menopausal symptoms such as hot flashes and vaginal dryness. Most postmenopausal women who take estrogen also take progestin (synthetic progesterone), because progestin negates the increased risk of uterine cancer in women taking estrogen alone. This combination is called hormone replacement therapy (HRT).

Estrogen improves both LDL and HDL cholesterol levels, so it was hoped that taking estrogen might reduce the risk of CHD. In addition, early findings suggested that HRT (usually 0.625 mg of Premarin daily) reduced the incidence of CHD events by as much as 50% in postmenopausal women. However, these findings were based on observational studies, and the women who chose to take HRT may simply have been healthier than the women who did not.

Then a randomized, controlled trial called the Heart and Estrogen/Progestin Replacement Study (HERS) found that the rates of heart attacks and death due to CHD were the same whether or not women took these hormones. More recently, an even larger randomized, controlled trial called the Women's Health Initiative found that after five years, women taking HRT (the study used Prempro) had a slightly increased risk of heart attacks, strokes, breast cancer, and blood clots in the lungs, compared with those taking a placebo. The HRT portion of the Women's Health Initiative study was halted, and experts now recommend that postmenopausal women not use HRT as a way to prevent CHD or CHD events such as heart attacks.

Women who have had a hysterectomy can take estrogen without progestin; this is called estrogen replacement therapy (ERT). A smaller portion of the Women's Health Initiative study involved assigning women to either estrogen alone or a placebo. This portion of the study is ongoing. It is possible that progestin may counteract the benefits of estrogen and that taking estrogen alone could have beneficial effects on the heart.

In the meantime, women who decide to take HRT to reduce the symptoms of menopause should limit the amount of time they use it. Women who have had breast cancer or have a family history of early breast cancer (a mother or sister who developed the disease before age 40) should be especially cautious about using HRT for any period of time. Such women may want to ask their doctor about tamoxifen (Nolvadex), which is often prescribed to prevent a recurrence in women with breast cancer and has beneficial effects on LDL and HDL cholesterol levels similar to those of estrogen.

Antianginal Drugs

The two goals in the treatment of angina symptoms are to decrease the heart's demand for oxygen and to increase its blood supply. Nitrates, beta-blockers, and calcium channel blockers are three types of drugs that can help control angina. (See the chart on pages 48–49.)

Nitrates. These drugs dilate both arteries and veins. Dilation of the coronary arteries increases blood flow to the heart; dilation of peripheral veins causes pooling of blood in the extremities. As a result, the heart has to pump less blood, and its workload and need for oxygen are reduced.

Sublingual nitroglycerin tablets (Nitrostat), which are placed under the tongue during an attack of angina, are the most common treatment to relieve angina pain. Translingual nitroglycerin spray (Nitrolingual), which is sprayed on or under the tongue, and sublingual isosorbide dinitrate tablets (Isordil) and chewable isosorbide dinitrate tablets are also effective. These four nitrates are fast acting and generally bring relief within two to three minutes. If five minutes pass without a reduction in symptoms, a second dose may be taken. If symptoms persist for another five minutes, a third dose may be recommended. But if symptoms persist for more than 15 minutes, they may be due to a heart attack rather than angina; call 911 and chew a regular-dose aspirin.

NEW RESEARCH

Aspirin Resistance Tied to Heart Attacks, Strokes

Doctors often recommend that people who've had a heart attack or ischemic stroke take a daily aspirin, which may prevent a second cardiovascular event by lowering the likelihood that platelets will form clots. Now, a study suggests that about 5% of people have platelets that do not respond to aspirin in the same way as they do in the the rest of the population. This group has an increased likelihood of experiencing a second heart attack or stroke even though they are on aspirin therapy.

The study enrolled 326 people, average age 60, with cardiovascular disease who were taking 325 mg of aspirin daily. About 5% of the participants were resistant to aspirin's antiplatelet effects. These people had nearly three times the risk of death, heart attack, or stroke over an average of 23 months than those who were responsive to aspirin (24% vs. 10%).

The test for aspirin resistance used in the study is not widely available, and currently there is no convenient, accurate way to determine who has aspirin resistance. But people who experience a heart attack or stroke while taking aspirin may be aspirin resistant and might benefit from another antiplatelet medication, such as clopidogrel (Plavix) or dipyridamole and aspirin (Aggrenox), according to an accompanying editorial.

JOURNAL OF THE AMERICAN COLLEGE OF CARDIOLOGY
Volume 41, pages 961 and 966
March 19, 2003

Antianginal Drugs 2004

Drug Type	Generic Name	Brand Name	Average Daily Dosage*	Wholesale Cost (Generic Cost)†
Beta-blockers	atenolol	Tenormin	50 to 100 mg	50 mg: $133 ($78)
	metoprolol	Lopressor	100 to 400 mg	100 mg: $137 ($76)
	extended-release	Toprol XL	up to 400 mg	100 mg: $114
	nadolol	Corgard	40 to 240 mg	80 mg: $263 ($140)
	propranolol	Inderal	80 to 320 mg	80 mg: $130 ($67)
	extended-release	Inderal LA	80 to 320 mg	80 mg: $149
Calcium channel blockers	amlodipine	Norvasc	2.5 to 10 mg	5 mg: $150
	diltiazem	Cardizem	90 to 240 mg	120 mg: $172 ($136)
	diltiazem, extended-release	Cardizem CD	180 to 240 mg	120 mg: $144 ($119)
		Cardizem SR	120 to 240 mg	120 mg: $163 ($113)
		Dilacor-XR	180 to 240 mg	120 mg: $146 ($119)
		Tiazac	120 to 240 mg	120 mg: $110 ($119)
	nicardipine	Cardene	60 mg	30 mg: $89 ($64)
	nifedipine, extended-release	Procardia XL	30 to 60 mg	30 mg: $157 ($116)
	verapamil	Calan	240 to 360 mg	120 mg: $99 ($43)
	verapamil, extended-release	Isoptin SR	240 to 360 mg	120 mg: $136 ($103)
Nitrates	**nitroglycerin**			
	For acute attacks:			
	sublingual tablets	Nitrostat	0.3 to 0.6 mg every 5 minutes; up to 3 tablets	0.3 mg: $10
	translingual spray	Nitrolingual	0.4 to 0.8 mg (1 to 2 sprays) every 5 minutes; up to 3 sets of sprays	0.4 mg, 30 sprays: $40
	For long-term management:			
	buccal tablets	Nitrogard	1 mg every 5 waking hours	2 mg: $48
	ointment	Nitro-Bid	1 to 2 inches (15 to 30 mg) every 6 to 8 hours	60 g: $16
	transdermal patches	Deponit	1 patch worn 12 hours a day (0.4 mg/hr)	30 patches: $58 ($68)
		Minitran		30 patches: $68 ($68)
		Nitro-Dur		30 patches: $64 ($68)
		Transderm-Nitro		30 patches: $59 ($68)
	isosorbide dinitrate	Isordil Titradose	80 to 160 mg	20 mg: $62 ($14)
	extended-release capsules	Dilatrate-SR	80 to 240 mg	40 mg: $78 ($62)
	sublingual tablets	Isordil	2.5 to 5 mg every 2 to 3 hours	10 mg: $40 ($10)
	chewable tablets	–	5 mg every 2 to 3 hours	(5 mg: $10)
	isosorbide mononitrate	ISMO	40 mg	20 mg: $94 ($70)
		Monoket	40 mg	20 mg: $109 ($70)
	extended-release tablets	IMDUR	30 to 120 mg	60 mg: $195 ($140)

How They Work	Advantages	Disadvantages
Beta-blockers slow the heart rate, lower blood pressure, and decrease the force of the heart's contractions; all of these effects reduce the heart's demand for oxygen. The slowed heart rate also prolongs the period of time between contractions, when most coronary blood flow occurs.	Beta-blockers decrease the risk of a second heart attack or death in people who have experienced a heart attack. These drugs also are effective for treating high blood pressure and some types of arrhythmias. Atenolol, nadolol, extended-release metoprolol, and extended-release propranolol need to be taken only once a day.	Side effects include fatigue, weakness, dizziness, decreased sexual function, vivid dreams, bronchospasm, and depression. These drugs should be avoided or used with caution in people with asthma, emphysema, peripheral vascular disease, diabetes, or a history of depression. Sudden withdrawal from beta-blocker therapy may worsen or induce angina or a heart attack; people who stop treatment with these drugs should do so gradually over several days.
Calcium channel blockers decrease the heart's demand for oxygen by reducing the heart rate, decreasing the force of the heart's contraction, and lowering blood pressure. They also increase blood flow through the coronary arteries, increasing the heart's oxygen supply. Verapamil and diltiazem reduce the increase in heart rate that occurs with exercise.	Calcium channel blockers also help to lower blood pressure. Side effects tend to be mild, except for patients with heart failure. Amlodipine and extended-release formulations of diltiazem, nifedipine, and verapamil need to be taken only once a day.	May cause headache, flushing, dizziness, nausea, or constipation. Legs and feet may become swollen (except with verapamil and diltiazem). Some of these drugs may aggravate heart failure or worsen certain arrhythmias.
Nitrates dilate the coronary arteries, increasing blood flow through these arteries to the oxygen-deprived areas of the heart. They also dilate the peripheral veins, causing blood to pool in the extremities. This effect decreases the amount of blood returned to the pumping chambers of the heart, which reduces the heart's workload and lessens its demand for oxygen.	Side effects are generally mild. Nitroglycerin can be used for treating or preventing acute attacks of angina and for day-to-day protection against angina. Comes in many forms: Tablets placed under the tongue (sublingual tablets) and aerosol spray administered on or under the tongue (translingual spray) are used to treat acute attacks; extended-release tablets, longer-acting tablets placed between the cheek and gum (buccal tablets), and ointments or transdermal patches applied directly on the skin provide continuous protection. Extended-release isosorbide dinitrate and isosorbide mononitrate are taken once or twice a day. Rotating the placement of transdermal patches prevents skin irritation.	Headaches are the most common side effect, but they usually decrease over time. Nausea and dizziness may occur and are worsened with alcohol use. If nitrates are constantly present in the bloodstream, drug tolerance develops and increasingly higher dosages are required to be effective. Thus, a daily drug-free interval (usually overnight) is advised to avoid tolerance. These drugs should be used with caution in people with glaucoma and hyperthyroidism.

* These dosages represent an average range for the prevention or treatment of angina. The precise effective dosage varies from patient to patient and depends on many factors. Do not make any changes in your medication without consulting your doctor.

† Average wholesale prices to pharmacists for 100 tablets or capsules (unless otherwise indicated) of the dosage strength listed. Costs to consumers are higher. If a generic version is available, the cost is listed in parentheses. Source: *Red Book, 2003* (Medical Economics Data, publishers).

Fast-acting nitrates may also prevent angina when taken shortly before beginning activities likely to provoke chest pain. Longer-acting medications, such as buccal nitroglycerin tablets (Nitrogard), which are held in the cheek, transdermal nitroglycerin patches (Deponit and other brands) and topical nitroglycerin ointments (Nitro-Bid), which are applied to the skin, and regular and extended-release isosorbide dinitrate (Isordil Titradose and Dilatrate-SR) and isosorbide mononitrate (ISMO, Monoket, and IMDUR) can provide protection against the onset of angina symptoms over the long term. But tolerance may develop with these longer-acting nitrates, and higher dosages may be needed to achieve the same effect. To prevent tolerance, longer-acting nitrates are discontinued for a period of time each day, usually overnight.

People may experience headaches when they first start to take nitrates, but this side effect tends to become less of a problem after a week or two. People who use nitrates should not take the erectile dysfunction drugs sildenafil (Viagra) or vardenafil (Levitra) because the combination may cause a dangerous drop in blood pressure. In addition, people should sit or lie down the first time they use nitrates in case they experience a drop in blood pressure.

For more information on the proper use of nitrates, see the feature on pages 52–53.

Beta-blockers. These drugs control angina by slowing heart rate and the force of the heart's contractions, thereby decreasing the workload and oxygen consumption of the heart. The slower heart rate also prolongs the time between contractions, allowing more blood to flow to the heart. Beta-blockers are also often prescribed to help prevent a second heart attack and improve survival in people who have had a heart attack. Common side effects of beta-blockers include fatigue, weakness, dizziness, decreased sexual function, vivid dreams, bronchospasm, and depression.

Calcium channel blockers. Like nitrates and beta-blockers, calcium channel blockers reduce the heart's workload, allow more blood to flow through the coronary arteries, and decrease the oxygen requirements of the heart muscle. These drugs can also alleviate angina caused by a spasm in a coronary artery. However, only the long-acting forms of calcium channel blockers should be used. Side effects of calcium channel blockers are usually mild and include headache, flushing, dizziness, nausea, fluid retention (edema), and constipation.

Combination therapy. In some people, neither beta-blockers nor calcium channel blockers alone provide sufficient relief of angina.

One study found that combining both types of drugs significantly lengthened the time individuals could exercise before experiencing angina.

TREATMENT OF ANGINA

When medication does not control angina pain, revascularization—bypass surgery or angioplasty—may be necessary. Since neither bypass surgery or angioplasty is a cure for atherosclerosis, it is essential to continue dietary and other preventive lifestyle measures and, in many cases, to take lipid-lowering drugs, blood pressure-lowering drugs, and aspirin after undergoing one of these procedures.

When angioplasty does not relieve angina pain or bypass surgery cannot be performed, another option called enhanced external counterpulsation may be tried.

Bypass Surgery

Each year in the United States, about 314,000 people undergo coronary artery bypass graft surgery (often called CABG or, simply, bypass surgery). During bypass surgery, a blood vessel from elsewhere in the body is used to reroute blood around a segment of a coronary artery narrowed by atherosclerosis. When needed, five or more bypass grafts can be performed during a single operation.

In most cases, at least one of the bypass grafts is constructed using an artery called the left internal mammary artery, or LIMA. This artery provides blood to the left side of the chest wall; it can be detached from the chest wall, with the open end sewn into the coronary artery beyond the blockage. Other bypass grafts may be constructed using a portion of a vein from the patient's leg. One end of the vein is sewn into the aorta near the heart, and the other end is attached to the coronary artery beyond the site of the blockage.

A LIMA graft usually lasts for 20 to 30 years, compared with about 10 years for a vein graft. In one study, a LIMA graft to the left anterior descending coronary artery was associated with a 27% lower risk of death than a vein graft to the same artery over a period of several years. A major reason for the better results with LIMA grafts is that they are less susceptible to the formation of new atherosclerosis compared with vein grafts. However, because it can take a long time to remove the LIMA, it may not be used in an emergency situation.

About 90% of people who undergo bypass surgery experience relief of angina symptoms after the procedure. Bypass surgery is an

Using Nitrate Medication To Manage Angina

Getting the most benefit from your nitrate medication with the fewest side effects requires carefully following your doctor's instructions.

If you suffer from angina, you are likely taking a nitrate to manage your condition. Nitrates are drugs that prevent and treat angina attacks by dilating the coronary arteries and peripheral veins. Dilation of the coronary arteries improves the supply of oxygen to the heart, while dilation of the peripheral veins reduces the heart's workload and thus its oxygen demand.

The three nitrate drugs for angina—nitroglycerin, isosorbide dinitrate, and isosorbide mononitrate—come in various formulations. Nitroglycerin is available as sublingual (held under the tongue) tablets, a translingual (on or under the tongue) spray, buccal (held in the cheek) tablets, a transdermal patch, and a topical ointment. Isosorbide dinitrate comes as sublingual tablets, chewable tablets, regular tablets, and extended-release capsules; isosorbide mononitrate comes in regular and extended-release tablets. The particular drug and formulation your doctor prescribes will depend in large part on the characteristics of your angina attacks (for example, how often they occur, when they occur, and what causes them).

Instructions for taking each of the nitrates and their formulations are outlined below. They may differ from those recommended by your doctor. To prevent a potentially fatal drop in blood pressure, never take sildenafil (Viagra) or vardenafil (Levitra) if you are on nitrate therapy.

Sublingual Nitroglycerin Tablets

Sublingual nitroglycerin (Nitrostat) is a fast-acting nitrate that is effective for relieving the pain of an angina attack or preventing an expected attack.

How to take. Sit down and place a sublingual nitroglycerin tablet under your tongue or between your cheek and gum. (Lie down if it is your first time taking sublingual nitroglycerin.) Allow the tablet to dissolve; be careful not to swallow it. If you take a sip of water before placing the tablet in your mouth, the medication will begin to work more quickly.

To relieve angina pain, take the tablet as soon as possible after the onset of symptoms. If symptoms are not relieved within five minutes, many doctors recommend taking another tablet. If symptoms are still present five minutes later, one more tablet may be taken. But if symptoms persist after taking three tablets in a 15-minute period, the symptoms may be due to a heart attack rather than to angina; call 911 and chew a regular-dose aspirin.

To prevent an expected attack, take one tablet five to ten minutes before an activity that produces angina symptoms.

Translingual Nitroglycerin Spray

Translingual nitroglycerin spray (Nitrolingual) acts rapidly and is used to relieve the pain of an angina attack or to prevent an expected attack.

How to take. Sit down and hold the spray container upright and near your mouth. Do not shake the container. Take a deep breath and spray the medication once or twice on or under your tongue. Close your mouth immediately and do not inhale or swallow the medication.

For relief of angina pain, use the spray as soon as possible after the onset of pain. If symptoms do not abate within five minutes, spray the medication on or under the tongue again. If necessary, repeat again after five minutes. If symptoms continue for more than 15 minutes despite three sets of sprays, you may be having a heart attack; call 911 and chew a regular-dose aspirin.

To prevent an expected attack, the spray should be used once five to ten minutes before an angina-producing activity.

Buccal Nitroglycerin Tablets

Buccal nitroglycerin tablets (Nitrogard) are rapid acting, but their effects last up to five hours. Therefore, it can be used not only for the treatment of angina pain and prevention of expected attacks, but also for general prevention of angina attacks over a longer period of time.

How to take. Place the tablet between the upper lip and gum or between the cheek and upper gum. Allow the tablet to dissolve; this should take about three to five hours. You should not chew or swallow the tablet during this time, but you can eat, drink, and talk while the tablet dissolves. If the tablet becomes dislodged, return it to its original position; if you accidentally swallow it, replace it with another.

To relieve angina pain, insert one tablet as soon as possible after the onset of symptoms. If symptoms do not disappear within five minutes, take a sublingual nitroglycerin tablet (see above) and contact your doctor.

To prevent an expected attack, use one tablet five to ten minutes before an angina-producing activity.

For the general prevention of angina, take a tablet every five hours while you are awake. Avoid falling asleep with the tablet in your mouth.

Transdermal Nitroglycerin Patch

Transdermal nitroglycerin patches (Deponit and other brands) are long-acting nitrates and are used for the general prevention of angina; the patches do not act fast enough to relieve symptoms of an ongoing attack or to prevent an expected attack.

How to take. Place the patch on a clean, dry area of skin that has little or no hair and is free of scars, cuts, and irritation. The best areas are on the chest, shoulders, upper arms, or back; do not use on the legs or lower arms. Wear the patch for 12 hours, then remove and discard. Apply a new patch only after a patch-free period (usually overnight). The patch-free period helps prevent drug tolerance (a reduced response to the drug over time). If skin around the patch becomes irritated, vary the site of patch application.

How To Store Nitrate Medication

Sublingual tablets, translingual sprays, and chewable tablets should be kept handy in case of an angina attack. For example, keep a supply in your bedroom, office, and coat or purse.

All nitrate medications should be stored at room temperature. Keep the medication away from hot, humid, or cold conditions, such as your car, bathroom, or refrigerator. Do not carry nitrates in an inside pocket, because the warmth of your body could cause the active ingredients to degrade.

Nitrates are also sensitive to light and oxygen, so be sure to keep the tablets and ointment in their original container with the cap tightly fastened, and the patches in their original pouches until ready to use. Sublingual tablets have a short shelf life and should be replaced every three to six months after the bottle is opened; other tablets should be replaced one year after opening the bottle. Sprays should be replaced after three years.

Topical Nitroglycerin Ointment

Topical nitroglycerin ointment (Nitro-Bid) is long acting and is used solely for the general prevention of angina attacks. It cannot relieve angina pain once it begins or prevent an expected attack of angina.

How to take. Squeeze the ointment in a thin, even layer onto the dose-measuring paper that comes with the ointment. Wipe the medication on an area of skin with little or no hair. The best areas are on the upper torso or arms. Do not rub or massage the ointment into the skin. In some cases, your doctor may instruct you to cover the ointment with a plastic wrap. Every six to eight hours remove any ointment residue and reapply the ointment. A 12-hour ointment-free period each day is recommended to prevent drug tolerance. To prevent irritation from the ointment, apply to a different spot each time.

Sublingual Isosorbide Dinitrate

Sublingual isosorbide dinitrate tablets (Isordil) are used for the relief of angina pain, the prevention of expected attacks, and the general prevention of attacks.

How to take. Sit down and place a tablet under your tongue or between your cheek and gum and let the tablet dissolve. Do not chew or swallow the tablet and try not to swallow too often until the tablet dissolves.

For the relief of angina pain, take immediately upon symptom onset. If pain is not relieved in five minutes, take a second tablet. If you are still experiencing pain five minutes later, take a third. If pain persists after three tablets in a 15-minute period, you may be having a heart attack; call 911 and chew a regular-dose aspirin.

For the prevention of expected angina attacks, take one tablet five to ten minutes before an activity that typically produces pain.

For general prevention of attacks, take a tablet every two to three hours while you are awake.

Chewable Isosorbide Dinitrate

Chewable isosorbide dinitrate tablets are used to relieve angina pain, prevent expected attacks, and prevent attacks over a longer period.

How to take. Sit down, then chew a tablet thoroughly and hold it in your mouth for one to two minutes before swallowing.

For relief of angina pain, take as soon as possible after symptom onset. If pain continues after five minutes, chew a second tablet. If pain is still present five minutes later, chew a third tablet. If chewing three tablets in 15 minutes does not produce pain relief, you may be having a heart attack; call 911 and chew a regular-dose aspirin.

For prevention of expected angina attacks, chew one tablet five to ten minutes before an activity that provokes angina.

For the general prevention of attacks, chew a tablet every two to three hours while you are awake.

Regular and Extended-release Isosorbide Dinitrate and Isosorbide Mononitrate

Regular isosorbide dinitrate (Isordil Titradose), extended-release isosorbide dinitrate (Dilatrate-SR), regular isosorbide mononitrate (ISMO, Monoket), and extended-release isosorbide mononitrate (IMDUR) are used only for the general prevention of angina attacks.

How to take. Swallow a tablet or capsule on an empty stomach (at least one hour before or two hours after a meal) with a full glass of water. Do not break, crush, or chew the extended-release tablets or capsules. Take regular isosorbide dinitrate three times a day with a 14-hour, tablet-free interval each day. Take regular isosorbide mononitrate twice a day; allow seven hours to elapse between the two doses. Extended-release isosorbide is taken once or twice a day.

extremely successful operation, even when the patient requires several bypass grafts, has extensive heart disease, or is elderly. Although a recent study found that people age 80 and older had a higher in-hospital death rate after bypass surgery than those under age 80 (8% vs. 3%), the benefits of bypass surgery may still outweigh the risks for many older people.

Despite the success of bypass surgery, the procedure is arduous for the patient. It requires general anesthesia and four to six days of hospitalization. The operation is usually performed with the help of a heart-lung machine that maintains blood circulation while the heart is stopped. Complications after surgery include heart attack (2% to 5%); stroke, memory loss, or confusion (6%); and infection (1% to 2%). Deaths due to the procedure occur less than 5% of the time, although the risk rises sharply when the patient's overall health is poor. Women used to be at higher risk from bypass surgery than men, but success rates for women appear to have caught up over the past few years, possibly because of an improved understanding of CHD in women.

Many of the problems encountered in bypass surgery can be traced to the need to stop the heart and place the patient on a heart-lung machine. Beating-heart bypass surgery, also known as off-pump bypass surgery, eliminates the need to stop the heart. To perform off-pump bypass surgery, surgeons use suction or compression to immobilize only a small portion of the heart. Studies suggest that the off-pump procedure is at least as effective as traditional bypass surgery and is associated with fewer immediate complications and no greater long-term risks. For more information on off-pump bypass surgery and how it compares to traditional bypass surgery, see the feature on pages 56–57.

Angioplasty

About 561,000 Americans a year undergo percutaneous transluminal coronary angioplasty (often called PTCA or, simply, angioplasty). Conventional angioplasty does not remove atherosclerotic plaque from the coronary arteries but instead widens the channel (lumen) through which blood flows by squeezing the plaque against the artery wall, cracking the hard part of the plaque, and/or stretching the artery. About 90% of people notice an immediate improvement in symptoms when the artery lumen is at least 50% open after angioplasty.

Angioplasty is performed in a cardiac catheterization laboratory and generally takes about one to two hours. It does not require general anesthesia and usually involves no more than a night's stay in the hospital. After the patient receives a sedative and local anesthesia to the groin area, a needle is inserted through a small incision into the femoral artery in the groin, and a plastic tube called a sheath is introduced. Then, a catheter is inserted through the sheath into the femoral artery. In some cases, the catheter is inserted into an artery in the forearm rather than in the groin.

The catheter is about a yard long and has an uninflated balloon at its tip. Guided by images on a screen, the cardiologist threads the catheter toward the heart and into the affected coronary artery. Guided by a thin wire inserted into the artery, the catheter is positioned so that the plaque straddles the balloon. The cardiologist then inflates the balloon several times, for 30 seconds to several minutes each time. After withdrawing the catheter, angiography is performed to assess the results.

In about 85% of cases, a small, scaffold-like device called a stent is permanently placed in the artery during angioplasty to help keep the artery open. Without stent implantation, the rate of restenosis (narrowing of the artery after angioplasty) ranges from 30% to 40%. Stent implantation reduces this rate to 10% to 20%. Potential problems are clot formation and tissue growth on the stent. The use of antiplatelet agents such as abciximab, eptifibatide, and tirofiban significantly decreases the risk of clots. Stents coated with substances that decrease clotting or smooth muscle cell proliferation are under study, and a stent coated with the antibiotic sirolimus was recently approved by the FDA (see the feature on pages 60–61). Other promising methods to reduce restenosis use slightly radioactive stents or irradiate the area around the stent.

The risks associated with angioplasty are low. Fewer than 1% of people die during the procedure. One possible complication during angioplasty is a total closure of the artery due to a clot, spasm, or tear in the artery wall. Closure of the artery can cause a heart attack (this occurs in about 2% to 4% of patients) or require emergency bypass surgery (in an additional 1% to 2% of patients). Because of this risk, people who require angioplasty in several vessels may need to recover for at least a day after the first angioplasty before the procedure is repeated on another vessel.

As might be expected, complication rates are lower when angioplasty is performed by more experienced physicians. One study found that a heart attack, emergency bypass surgery, or death occurred in 9% of angioplasty patients whose doctors performed 70 or fewer procedures annually, compared with only 3% of patients

NEW RESEARCH

Where Should You Have Bypass Surgery?

Although many researchers study the death rate during or just after bypass surgery to measure quality of care at different hospitals, new research shows that the rate of hospital readmission is an additional, effective way to make this determination.

Investigators analyzed data from 16,325 patients who underwent bypass surgery in New York in 1999. Within 30 days of the procedure, 2,111 (13%) were readmitted to the hospital because of complications. Two factors increased the readmission rates: having a surgeon who performed fewer than 100 bypass surgeries per year and having the procedure at a hospital with a high death rate for bypass surgery.

Infection (28%), heart failure (16%), heart attack or poor blood flow to the heart (8%), and arrhythmias (8%) were the most common reasons for readmission. Rates of readmission increased with age and were higher for women than for men; they were also higher in blacks than in other races. Patients admitted to a nursing home after the bypass procedure and those who needed to stay in the hospital for five days or longer after the procedure also had increased rates of readmission.

JOURNAL OF THE AMERICAN MEDICAL ASSOCIATION
Volume 290, page 773
August 13, 2003

A New Technique for Bypass Surgery

The off-pump procedure lets surgeons restore blood flow to the heart while it is still beating and may reduce complications associated with traditional bypass.

Bypass surgery is a common treatment for blockages in the coronary arteries. The procedure involves taking a blood vessel (the left internal mammary artery from the chest or a portion of a vein from the leg) and using it to reroute blood flow to the heart, thereby "bypassing" narrowed coronary arteries. By restoring adequate circulation to blood-starved areas of the heart muscle, bypass surgery provides relief from angina and, in some people, reduces the risk of heart attack and death.

Traditionally, the procedure is performed through an open incision in the sternum, or breastbone. Medication is administered to stop the heart, and the patient is temporarily placed on a heart-lung machine, which does the work of the heart and lungs.

Unfortunately, this procedure is associated with risks, including serious bleeding, stroke, and kidney failure. In addition, contact between the patient's blood and the artificial surfaces of the machine can cause inflammation throughout the body that can damage multiple organs. The heart-lung procedure may also contribute to the cognitive decline that some people experience following bypass surgery. However, it's now possible to perform bypass surgery on a beating heart, eliminating the need to stop the heart and use the heart-lung machine.

Beating-heart bypass, also known as off-pump bypass, has been in routine use for only a few years. Like traditional bypass surgery, an incision is made in the sternum, and a blood vessel from the chest or leg is used to bypass a blocked coronary artery. However, in the off-pump procedure, surgeons use suction or compression to immobilize only a small portion of the heart. Consequently, the heart can continue to pump blood to the rest of the body, and the surgeon can bypass as many diseased arteries as necessary.

According to the National Center for Health Statistics, more than 300,000 people have heart bypass surgery each year in the United States. Experts estimate that about one third of these procedures are performed on a beating heart and that an additional 20% of patients will likely have an off-pump bypass as more surgeons learn the technique and the procedure becomes more widely available.

Comparing Outcomes

Off-pump bypass appears to be at least as effective as on-pump bypass in many patients. A 2003 study in *The New England Journal of Medicine* reported that 139 patients who had traditional bypass and 142 who had off-pump bypass had nearly the same rates of death, stroke, heart attack, and repeat bypass surgery or angioplasty one year later.

The issue, then, is whether off-pump bypass can avert some of the complications associated with traditional bypass surgery. Early findings are encouraging. When off-pump bypass surgery is appropriate, it has at least three significant advantages over traditional surgery. First, it is associated with less neurological injury, most of which is related to the use of the heart-lung machine itself. Second, patients do not require as many blood transfusions. Third, patients retain less fluid after surgery, so they can be discharged from the hospital and resume their normal activities sooner.

Additional research suggests that off-pump bypass may be associated with a reduced risk of other complications compared with traditional bypass surgery:

Stroke risk. It has been estimated that about 3% of patients who undergo traditional bypass suffer a stroke, but some research indicates a lower risk of stroke in carefully selected patients who have beating-heart bypass surgery. In a 2002 study in *The Annals of Thoracic Surgery*, researchers compared outcomes in 2,320 off-pump bypass patients and 8,069 traditional bypass patients. Although stroke risk was low in both groups, patients undergoing traditional bypass surgery were almost twice as likely to suffer a postoperative stroke as patients who had off-pump surgery.

Cognitive function. According to the findings of a recent study in *The New England Journal of Medicine*, traditional bypass surgery is associated with a decline in cognitive function that may persist for years. About half of patients experience short-term memory loss right after the traditional procedure, and 40% of traditional bypass patients show some degree of mental impairment five years later. It is not known whether some of these patients might have experienced cognitive decline over the five-year period, even if they had not had the bypass surgery.

Efforts to determine whether the beating-heart bypass procedure can decrease the likelihood of cognitive decline after bypass surgery have yielded inconsistent results. Dutch researchers reported in the *Journal of the American Medical Association* in 2002 that patients undergoing off-pump surgery had better cognitive function three months after the surgery than did those undergoing traditional bypass. However, the differences in cognitive function between the two groups declined over time and became negligible after one year. A larger study is needed to demonstrate whether there are any long-term cognitive benefits of off-pump surgery.

Kidney function. Another recent study in *The Annals of Thoracic Surgery* found that patients with kidney problems were more likely to develop acute kidney failure and experience stroke or blood loss after traditional bypass surgery than after the off-pump procedure.

High-risk patients. Some people, such as those who are overweight or older than 80 years of age, are at increased risk for complications from bypass surgery. Some research suggests that these people may also benefit from off-pump bypass. A 2002 study in *Circulation* reported the results of 4,321 bypass procedures, many in overweight patients. More than 75% of the patients underwent off-pump bypass surgery, and these individuals had a reduced risk of death, spent less time in intensive care, needed fewer blood transfusions, and had a lower risk of stroke than the traditional bypass patients. Another study, also in *Circulation*, reported similar benefits of off-pump bypass compared with traditional bypass in 125 people over age 80.

Should You Have Off-Pump Bypass?

Although many bypass patients may benefit from off-pump surgery, some are better candidates for traditional bypass surgery. These people include patients with extremely small or very narrow blood vessels, those whose coronary arteries are not easily accessible, and people with severe left ventricular dysfunction. For these individuals, the surgeon may be better able to access their arteries with traditional rather than off-pump bypass surgery.

There is some concern that off-pump bypass surgery may not restore blood flow as completely as traditional bypass in some patients. In addition, researchers are working on ways to make both procedures safer and more effective. Some of these improvements include changes to the heart-lung machine, devices to trap microemboli (tiny fat particles that can enter the bloodstream during bypass surgery and travel to the brain), and different ways to stabilize the heart during off-pump surgery.

If you are interested in off-pump bypass, make sure your surgeon is familiar with the procedure. Also, keep in mind that your surgeon may not decide whether to do an off-pump or traditional procedure until the time of surgery, when the condition of your heart and arteries is more apparent. In case the surgeon needs to switch to a traditional bypass during the procedure, a specialist (called a perfusionist) who is trained in operating the heart-lung machine is always present.

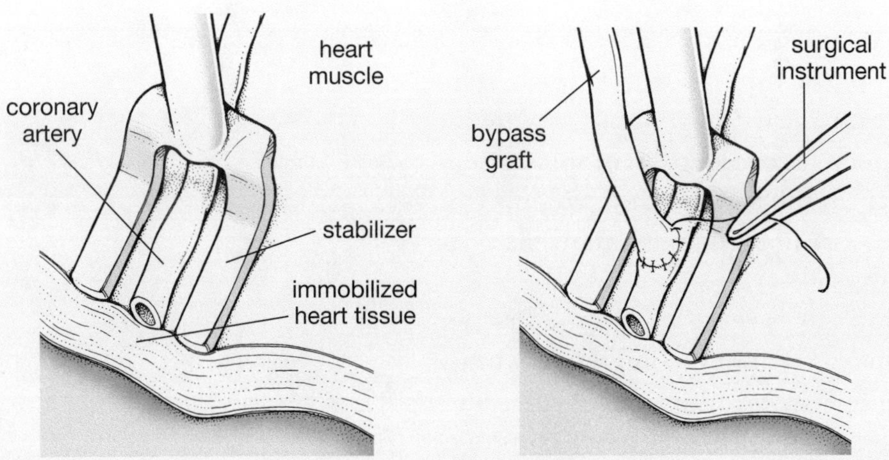

Off-Pump Bypass Surgery

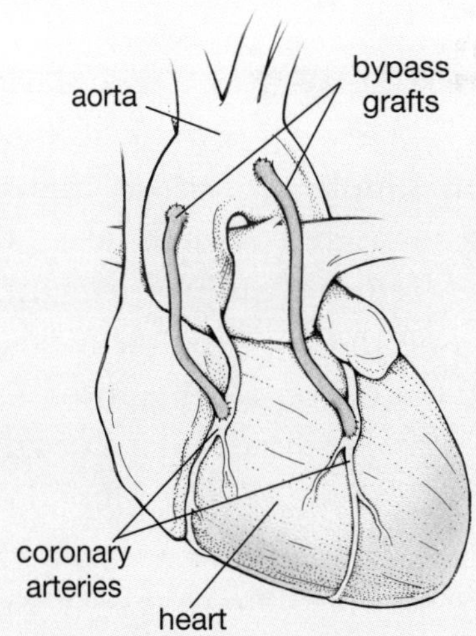

The Heart After Bypass

whose doctors performed more than 270 procedures annually. But the complication rate depends on many factors, and physicians who perform fewer angioplasties can still have low complication rates by performing the procedure only on patients at low risk for complications.

Other Procedures To Improve Blood Supply to the Heart

Besides bypass surgery and angioplasty, other procedures such as atherectomy and laser ablation are used in certain circumstances to improve blood flow through the coronary arteries.

Atherectomy. This procedure uses a high-speed rotary blade or drill to shave away portions of plaque narrowing a coronary artery. The blade or drill is delivered to the site of arterial blockage using a catheter. Atherectomy appears to be most successful when performed on large, straight arteries. The blade is usually the device of choice for plaque limited to one side of the artery wall; the drill typically yields better results than angioplasty for very long obstructions.

Laser ablation. This procedure resembles angioplasty except that the balloon is replaced with a probe. The probe is heated with a beam of laser light to cut through the plaque blocking the coronary artery. A potential complication of laser ablation is creating a hole in the artery wall. The procedure may eventually prove useful in reopening completely blocked arteries, as well as in destroying plaques that cannot be treated with angioplasty because they are too long or hardened by calcium deposits.

Bypass Surgery vs. Angioplasty

Angioplasty has several advantages over bypass surgery. It is a relatively simple procedure, there is no need for general anesthesia, and the rigors of open heart surgery are avoided. Angioplasty generally requires only a one-night stay in the hospital and patients can resume their normal activities almost immediately. Angioplasty is also less expensive than bypass surgery.

A major disadvantage of angioplasty is restenosis in the first six months after the procedure. People who undergo angioplasty must accept the risk that a repeat angioplasty or, ultimately, bypass surgery may become necessary. Recurring angina is another consideration. These risks are considerably decreased with stent implantation. Another disadvantage is that many people with CHD are not suitable candidates for angioplasty.

Bypass surgery may keep arteries open longer and improve blood flow through the coronary arteries more than angioplasty.

Bypass surgery generally provides good relief of angina for at least five years. In addition, bypass surgery is generally favored over angioplasty in people with one or more of the following:

Disease in the left main coronary artery. This vessel is the main artery supplying blood to the heart, and even a brief period of blockage could damage heart muscle or be fatal.

Diffuse CHD. Angioplasty is not effective for the treatment of multiple blockages in several vessels.

Blockages at an arterial branch. If the blockage is at a point where one artery meets another, angioplasty may move the plaque into the adjacent artery, causing a new blockage.

Diabetes. In the Bypass Angioplasty Revascularization Investigation (BARI) study, seven-year survival for people with diabetes was significantly better in those who underwent bypass surgery (76%) than angioplasty (56%).

Other factors. Other factors that make bypass surgery a better choice than angioplasty include severe disease of the three major coronary arteries (especially in people with reduced left ventricular function) and a history of heart failure.

Two drawbacks to bypass surgery are longer hospital stays and rehabilitation time than with angioplasty. In addition, a recent study of 261 bypass surgery patients found that about 40% of them had a decline in cognitive function that persisted five years after surgery. It is possible, however, that this decline was caused by underlying vascular disease and not the surgery itself.

Enhanced External Counterpulsation

Some people with angina do not obtain complete pain relief from medications or angioplasty and cannot undergo bypass surgery because of poor health. For these people, a procedure called enhanced external counterpulsation (EECP) may improve angina symptoms and quality of life.

In EECP, the person lies on a table and inflatable cuffs are placed around the calves, lower thighs, and upper thighs of each leg. The cuffs are rapidly inflated in sequential order beginning with the cuffs at the calves and working upward. Cuff inflation is timed so that it occurs when the heart is at rest (that is, when the heart muscle is receiving oxygen-rich blood from the coronary arteries). Cuff deflation coincides with the heart's contractions (that is, when oxygenated blood is pumped to the rest of the body). EECP is an outpatient procedure and typically requires 35 sessions over a period of six to seven weeks. Each EECP session takes about an hour.

NEW RESEARCH

Gene Therapy During Angioplasty Improves Blood Flow

Preliminary research indicates that a type of gene therapy performed during angioplasty may improve blood flow to the heart better than angioplasty alone.

The research involved 103 Finns with CHD who were randomized to undergo angioplasty with or without gene therapy. The gene increases levels of vascular endothelial growth factor (VEGF), which stimulates the repair of damaged blood vessels and the growth of new blood vessels, especially in tissue receiving inadequate oxygen. The gene was delivered to the target artery in an inactivated virus or in liposomes made of synthetic fat molecules.

After six months, the rate of restenosis was about the same in all the participants. However, the virus-treated group had significantly improved blood flow to the heart compared with the liposome-treated or angioplasty-alone group. Side effects of gene treatment included fever. One patient in the virus group died of a previously undetected aortic aneurysm, and two new cancers developed in the liposome group. A safety monitoring board concluded that gene therapy did not cause these three events.

According to an accompanying editorial, this therapy, currently in phase 2 trials, is unique because it recruits the body's natural ability to heal itself.

CIRCULATION
Volume 107, pages 2635 and 2677
June 3, 2003

The New Drug-Coated Stent

The Cypher stent dramatically reduces the chance of arterial narrowing after successful angioplasty.

Angioplasty is an effective treatment to widen coronary arteries narrowed by atherosclerosis. But the effectiveness of angioplasty is limited by restenosis, in which the treated artery narrows over time. In 1993, doctors began to address this problem by placing a stent in the coronary artery during the angioplasty procedure. Without a stent, restenosis occurs in up to 40% of angioplasties; the rate decreases to 10% to 20% with a stent.

But stents are prone to tissue overgrowth and clot formation, both of which narrow the artery and can lead to heart attacks. So researchers began to coat stents with the anticoagulant drug heparin in an effort to reduce the risk of clots. Then in 2003, the U.S. Food and Drug Administration (FDA) approved the Cypher stent, a far more effective stent coated with a drug that inhibits the overgrowth of tissue.

Preventing Restenosis

A stent is a stainless steel, scaffold-like device that is permanently implanted in the portion of the artery opened during angioplasty. Some tissue usually grows over the stent; excessive tissue growth can lead to restenosis.

The Cypher stent is coated with sirolimus, an antibiotic that the FDA originally approved in 1999 to prevent rejection of kidney transplants. The drug has antifungal, immunosuppressive, anti-inflammatory, and anti-cell-division actions, each of which may contribute to its ability to prevent restenosis.

Heparin-coated stents release little of the drug, but the Cypher stent is designed to release (or "elute") the drug slowly over several weeks. About 80% of the sirolimus is released in the first 28 days after stent implantation, when smooth muscle cell migration and proliferation are most likely to occur.

The Evidence

The most impressive evidence for the Cypher stent comes from a study published in 2002 in *The New England Journal of Medicine*. The study randomized 238 people with angina to receive either the Cypher stent or a standard, uncoated stent. After six months, the size of the opening in the artery (lumen) with the Cypher stent was the same as it was just after angioplasty. But with the standard stent, the lumen was 0.8 mm smaller in diameter than it was initially. Also, at six months, no patient with the Cypher stent had restenosis (defined as more than a 50% reduction in the lumen), compared with 27% of patients with the standard stent. After one year, only 6% of the Cypher patients experienced a major cardiac event (death,

Researchers are uncertain why EECP works. One possibility is that it stimulates the growth of tiny coronary blood vessels that help "bypass" the blocked vessels, thereby increasing blood flow and oxygen to areas of the heart that were previously receiving insufficient amounts.

People with uncontrolled heart failure, very high blood pressure, a heart rate higher than 120 beats per minute, lung disease, or a history of phlebitis (vein inflammation) should not undergo EECP.

TREATMENT OF UNSTABLE ANGINA

An episode of unstable angina is an emergency situation that often requires hospitalization. At the hospital, the patient will likely be given intravenous heparin along with aspirin to inhibit further clot formation. Intravenous nitroglycerin is also given to help dilate the coronary arteries. Thrombolytic—or clot-busting—therapy usually is not used because the blood clots involved in this type of angina do not respond to this therapy.

heart attack, repeat angioplasty, or bypass operation), compared with 29% of the standard-stent patients.

Further benefits of the Cypher stent were reported in October 2003 in *The New England Journal of Medicine*. In this study, 1,058 people with coronary heart disease were randomized to receive either the Cypher stent or a standard, uncoated stent. After about nine months, people who received the Cypher stent were significantly less likely to die from coronary heart disease, have a heart attack, or need angioplasty or bypass surgery than those who received a standard stent (9% vs. 21%).

Drawbacks

The Cypher stent has some limitations. A letter issued by the FDA on October 29, 2003 warned physicians about a rare but potential risk of clot formation associated with the Cypher stent. Of the hundreds of thousands of patients who had received the stent at the time the letter was issued, the FDA said it had received 290 reports of clots occurring within 30 days of implantation of the stent, including more than 60 deaths.

Other complications associated with implantation of the Cypher stent include fever, bleeding in the groin at the incision site for the angioplasty, chest pain, irregular heart rhythm, emergency bypass surgery, and stroke. Many of these occur after implantation of an uncoated stent as well. Because only tiny amounts of sirolimus are released into the blood, side effects from the sirolimus itself are rare but can include fatigue, joint pain, diarrhea, infection, and tumor formation.

Also, the Cypher device is not appropriate for all people who undergo angioplasty. Patients who are allergic to stainless steel, plastics, or sirolimus should not undergo implantation of this stent, nor should patients who are unable to take the anticoagulant or antiplatelet drugs that are needed after the procedure.

Further, some questions about the Cypher stent can only be answered with more study and experience with the device. First, researchers are uncertain about the benefits and risks of the stent beyond one year of implantation. Second, no one is sure if the same degree of benefit seen in the clinical trials (which studied only a very narrow patient population) will be true for the general population.

The last unanswered question is whether the device will prove to be cost effective. Each Cypher stent can cost up to $3,500, which is considerably more than the cost of a standard stent ($700 to $800), and often more than one stent is placed. Over the long term, however, costs will likely be lower for the Cypher stent because patients should require fewer repeat angioplasties and bypass surgeries—but this still needs to be determined.

Researchers are also testing stents coated with agents such as paclitaxel (an anticancer drug), everolimus (a synthetic analogue of sirolimus), and two immunosuppressive agents, tacrolimus and mycophenolic acid.

After unstable angina is brought under control at the hospital, the next step is to determine how to manage the condition over the long term. The doctor makes this decision based on the severity of the condition and the response to initial treatment in the hospital. If patients respond initially to heparin and aspirin and are at relatively low risk for a heart attack, they can be treated with medication. Treatment with medication involves long-term aspirin and, sometimes, clopidogrel to inhibit blood clotting, nitrates to widen blood vessels, and beta-blockers to decrease the workload of the heart.

Individuals at intermediate or high risk for a heart attack will most likely undergo coronary angiography (see page 26) to determine the extent and location of the blockage(s). Patients are at high risk for a heart attack if they do not respond to in-hospital treatment with medication or have a history of angioplasty or bypass surgery, heart failure, a low ejection fraction, or ventricular arrhythmias. The angiography results help the doctor determine whether these patients can be managed with medication or will require angioplasty or bypass surgery.

Angioplasty or bypass surgery also may be performed if medication fails to prevent subsequent episodes of unstable angina. When angioplasty or bypass surgery is performed for unstable angina, a balloon may be placed in the aorta prior to the procedure. The balloon is inflated and deflated to increase blood flow to the coronary arteries when the heart is at rest between beats.

TREATMENT OF HEART ATTACK

Treatment of a heart attack often begins in the ambulance while the patient is being transported to the hospital. Paramedics can administer oxygen, provide nitrates and aspirin, begin cardiopulmonary resuscitation (CPR) in the event of a cardiac arrest, and treat arrhythmias. At the hospital, heart attack patients are taken to the coronary care unit. Morphine is commonly given to relieve pain, sedate the patient, and reduce the heart's need for oxygen. The patient is attached to an ECG monitor to detect arrhythmias that may require immediate treatment.

Thrombolytic Therapy

When a diagnosis of a heart attack is made early, usually within 12 hours of the onset of symptoms, an injection of streptokinase or tissue-type plasminogen activator (t-PA) will often open a blocked coronary artery by dissolving the blood clot that is impeding the flow of blood. Controlled studies show that such thrombolytic (clot-dissolving) therapy can restore blood flow through the blocked artery, reduce the amount of damage to the heart muscle, and improve survival after a heart attack in many patients. Drawbacks of thrombolytic therapy include a failure to open the artery in about 20% of patients and serious bleeding, especially in the brain, in less than 5% of patients. If thrombolytic therapy fails to reopen the blocked artery, emergency angioplasty or bypass surgery may be carried out.

Aspirin and intravenous heparin are usually administered after thrombolytic therapy to reduce the likelihood of further clot formation. Heparin is generally continued for 24 to 48 hours, and a daily aspirin is taken indefinitely thereafter.

Emergency Angioplasty/Bypass Surgery

Several recent studies have compared thrombolytic therapy with angioplasty in the period immediately following a heart attack. The blocked artery was more likely to remain open in people who underwent angioplasty than in those who received thrombolytic therapy. Although emergency angioplasty was no more effective than thrombolytic therapy in preventing damage to the heart muscle, angioplasty was better at preventing recurrent ischemia, another heart attack, and death.

Emergency angioplasty is probably preferable to thrombolytic therapy for those at highest risk for death—people older than age 75 and those with damage to the front portion of the heart or sustained low blood pressure. Emergency bypass surgery is considered when thrombolytic treatment has not succeeded and coronary angiography shows that the blockages cannot be treated effectively with angioplasty.

Risk Stratification

Early in their hospital stay, heart attack patients should be "risk stratified," which means that they should undergo tests to assess their risk of future CHD events. The results of these tests help doctors determine whether angioplasty or bypass surgery is needed. Coronary angiography is commonly used for risk stratification. Assessment of left ventricular function by echocardiography or during angiography also is important in risk stratification. In some cases of mild heart attacks with no apparent complications, or when angiography is not appropriate, a low-level exercise stress test is carried out five to seven days after the heart attack.

Recovery

If recovery from a heart attack is uneventful and angioplasty or bypass surgery is not necessary, patients are usually discharged from the hospital after a week or less. Activities are slowly increased over the next eight weeks or so, and resumption of a full schedule is usually possible about two months after leaving the hospital.

Heart attack patients with significant damage to the front wall of the left ventricle often are treated with warfarin in an effort to prevent the formation of blood clots. A blood clot that detaches from the heart and travels through the circulatory system can cause a stroke if it blocks a blood vessel to the brain. (About 5% of heart attack patients suffer a stroke.) All patients who can take beta-blockers should begin long-term treatment with these drugs after a heart attack. Many patients benefit from taking an ACE inhibitor and a statin over the long term as well.

NEW RESEARCH

Even If Delayed, Angioplasty May Be Better Than Drugs After Heart Attack

While angioplasty is generally a better treatment than thrombolytic (clot-busting) drugs for a heart attack, patients may receive thrombolytic therapy if the nearest hospital does not perform angioplasty. However, a new study shows that even when patients have to wait to be transferred to a facility that performs angioplasty, angioplasty may still be a better option.

Researchers studied 1,572 people who had a heart attack; some were taken to hospitals that did not perform angioplasty, others to hospitals that did perform angioplasty. The participants were randomized to receive either thrombolytic therapy or angioplasty. When patients randomized to angioplasty were taken initially to a hospital that didn't perform the procedure, they were transferred within three hours to a facility that could perform one.

Patients who received angioplasty were 75% less likely to have another heart attack in the next 30 days than those who received thrombolytic therapy (1.6% vs. 6.3%); this relationship held even when people who needed to be transferred to another hospital to undergo angioplasty were compared with those who received immediate thrombolytic therapy (1.9% vs. 6.2%). Optimally, the transfer should be within two hours, the authors note.

THE NEW ENGLAND JOURNAL OF MEDICINE
Volume 349, page 733
August 21, 2003

Restoring Hearts With Cell Transplants

Researchers are investigating whether muscle and bone marrow cells can help regenerate heart tissue damaged by a heart attack.

Thanks to treatments such as clot-busting drugs, angioplasty, and bypass surgery, more Americans are surviving heart attacks than ever before. Unfortunately, none of these treatments repairs the heart muscle damage caused by a heart attack. This damage leads to heart failure in up to 30% of heart attack patients. Heart transplantation is a potential treatment for heart failure, but the scarcity of donor organs and the potential for organ rejection limit its usefulness. In addition, the five-year death rate for heart transplantation is about 30%.

Unlike some other tissues, heart muscle is generally thought to be incapable of regenerating itself after an injury, but researchers are investigating new ways of helping the heart to heal. One important area of research involves transplanting cells from other areas of the body into the heart to see whether these cells can spur tissue growth in areas damaged by a heart attack.

Using the Body's Own Cells
Myoblasts from skeletal muscle and cells from bone marrow are being examined for their ability to replace damaged heart muscle. Myoblasts are cells found in muscle tissue that are able to form new cells that turn into muscle cells; bone marrow cells have not yet committed to form into any particular type of tissue and are able to replicate many times and differentiate into specialized cells.

Myoblasts and bone marrow cells can be taken from the patient's own body—rather than from an embryo—and grown in a lab. When introduced into the heart, the myoblasts may multiply and grow new muscle cells, while some bone marrow cells may develop into heart muscle cells—and form new blood vessels as well.

It's too early to say which type of cell, if any, will be most effective in treating patients with heart failure. It's possible that muscle cells might help the heart pump more strongly, and bone marrow cells might help grow new blood vessels in the heart. Perhaps a combination of the two would be best. For now, though, bone marrow cells are the main focus of research.

Recent Research
Research into cell transplantation for heart patients is in its infancy. Though the research has several limitations—the studies have included only a small number of participants, and very few have included a control group—the technique shows promise.

In one trial of 10 patients, published in 2003, thigh-muscle cells were implanted during bypass surgery into scar tissue caused by a heart attack. Eleven months after the procedure, the patients had some improvement in heart function. In another study also published in 2003, German doctors implanted bone marrow cells into the hearts of six heart attack survivors during bypass surgery; four had improved heart function,

TREATMENT OF COMPLICATIONS OF A HEART ATTACK

Complications are most likely to occur when a heart attack is severe. The most common complications of a heart attack are heart failure and arrhythmias. Other possibilities include severe dysfunction of the mitral valve (the valve that prevents blood from flowing back from the left ventricle to the left atrium and lungs) due to rupture of the muscles that hold the two segments of the valve in place; rupture of the wall that separates the left ventricle from the right ventricle; rupture of the outside wall of the left ventricle (which is almost always immediately fatal); a ballooning of the wall of the left ventricle (ventricular aneurysm) due to scar tissue formation; and emboli to vital organs such as the brain, legs, or kidneys.

and five had significantly improved blood flow to the heart. However, because the participants in both of these studies also had bypass surgery, it is not clear which procedure produced the improvement.

Recently, doctors from Hong Kong used a catheter inserted in the femoral artery to implant bone marrow cells into the hearts of eight patients with angina that did not respond to drug treatment. After three months, angina symptoms and blood flow to the heart had improved. In another recent study, researchers used a catheter to implant bone marrow cells into 14 Brazilian heart failure patients. At two and four months after the treatment, patients showed less symptoms of heart failure and their hearts had improved pumping ability compared with seven other patients who did not receive the treatment.

Though cell transplantation appears to improve heart function, it has been difficult to show whether transplanted cells are converted into heart muscle cells. However, two recent findings suggest that the transplanted cells undergo some sort of transformation. First, an autopsy of a man who had muscle stem cells injected into his heart showed that the transplanted cells had matured and were slightly different from regular skeletal muscle cells. Second, autopsies of four women who received bone marrow transplants from men (as a treatment for leukemia) showed that a small percentage of their heart muscle cells contained male genetic material—suggesting that transplanted bone marrow cells are capable of becoming heart muscle cells. Researchers are working on a way to mark the transplanted cells so that they can be distinguished from already existing heart tissue.

Possible Complications

One complication that has been associated with cell transplantation in several studies is significant and potentially dangerous arrhythmias (irregular heart rhythms), although it's not clear whether the cell transplant was the cause. No other serious complications have been reported. However, it's not known whether some transplanted cells might grow into scar tissue or a tumor instead of becoming heart muscle or new blood vessels.

Further Investigation

Cardiac cell transplantation sounds promising, and it has the potential to help heart failure patients who might otherwise have to undergo a heart transplant or who have no other option. However, the effectiveness of the procedure is not proven, and no one knows how long any benefits might last. It's also not known when cell transplantation might be most effective: immediately after a heart attack or at a later time.

A randomized clinical trial currently under way in Europe should help provide some answers. In the trial, several hundred heart attack survivors with blocked coronary arteries will have some of their own bone marrow cells infused into their coronary arteries. The other half of the participants will serve as a control group, having some of their bone marrow cells removed but receiving an infusion that doesn't contain any of these cells.

If you are interested in participating in a trial of cell transplantation, you can visit one of the following Web sites to learn whether the procedure is being investigated in your area: www.clinicaltrials.gov; www.centerwatch.com; and www.trialscentral.org.

Heart Failure

The first steps in the treatment of acute heart failure, in which fluid builds up in the lungs (pulmonary edema), are bed rest, oxygen supplementation, and intravenous administration of morphine, nitrates, and diuretics until the condition stabilizes. Angioplasty or bypass surgery may be performed if heart failure is due to low blood flow to the heart and if greater blood flow would improve the function of the heart muscle. Sometimes a poor response to these treatments is due to damage to the mitral valve or its supporting structures, causing blood to back up into the lungs. Correction of this condition may require surgical repair of the valve or replacement of the valve with an artificial one.

Guidelines developed by the Agency for Health Care Policy and Research for managing chronic heart failure are as follows:

- Left ventricular function should be measured in all people who have symptoms strongly suggestive of heart failure;

- People with moderate to severe left ventricular dysfunction should be treated with an ACE inhibitor even if they have no symptoms of heart failure. Most people with established heart failure should be treated with an ACE inhibitor, a diuretic, and, sometimes, digoxin (Lanoxin). ACE inhibitors tend to be underused and prescribed at too low a dose, possibly because of concerns about their side effects;
- Those with angina or a previous heart attack should be assessed to determine whether they would benefit from angioplasty or bypass surgery;
- Sodium intake should be restricted to 2,000 mg or less a day to help control fluid accumulation;
- Alcohol should be avoided;
- Regular exercise may help prevent symptoms of heart failure from worsening; and
- Patients should report to their doctor any weight gain of more than 3 lbs. per week because rapid weight gain may indicate excessive fluid retention. Any new symptoms or worsening of previous symptoms also should be reported.
- Patients with severe chronic heart failure should limit their activities and plan periodic rest sessions.

Diuretics and digoxin have been used to treat heart failure for many years. Although thiazide diuretics are effective for mild heart failure, more potent agents, such as the loop diuretic furosemide (Lasix), are used for severe fluid retention. The Randomized Aldactone Evaluation Study (RALES) showed that, compared with a placebo, 25 mg daily of the potassium-sparing diuretic spironolactone (Aldactone) substantially reduced heart failure symptoms, hospitalizations for heart failure, and overall risk of death over a two-year period in people with severe heart failure. Patients whose heart failure does not respond to treatment may require a combination of several types of diuretic drugs, each with a different mechanism of action.

Addition of a beta-blocker to the standard drug treatment of a diuretic and an ACE inhibitor also is successful in many patients. In a meta-analysis of 17 studies, the risk of death from all causes was 31% lower in heart failure patients treated with beta-blockers than in those not receiving a beta-blocker. The beta-blockers carvedilol (Coreg), metoprolol (Lopressor), and extended-release metoprolol (Toprol XL) are approved by the FDA for mild to moderate (class II or III) heart failure. In three other large clinical trials,

NEW RESEARCH

Beta-Blocker Appears Safe, Effective Early in Heart Failure Treatment

Although beta-blockers benefit many patients with heart failure, they are generally underused, possibly because of concerns that they may be risky at first and that benefits may not appear for some time. Yet a recent study finds that the risk of starting treatment is minimal and that probable benefits occur within the first few weeks of treatment.

In the study, 2,289 people with heart failure were randomized to take the beta-blocker carvedilol (Coreg) or a placebo. All patients also received other standard medications for heart failure.

Worsening of heart failure in the first eight weeks was no more likely with carvedilol than the placebo (5% vs. 6%). (However, dizziness, low blood pressure, swelling from fluid buildup, and a slowed heart rate were more common with carvedilol.) During this period, the carvedilol group showed a statistically nonsignificant reduction in deaths, hospitalizations, and treatment stoppages. These probable benefits appeared within the first two to three weeks. In a previous analysis of these same patients, carvedilol lowered the death rate by 35% over 10 months compared with the placebo.

An accompanying editorial urges physicians to seriously consider prescribing these drugs to most heart failure patients.

JOURNAL OF THE AMERICAN MEDICAL ASSOCIATION
Volume 289, pages 712 and 754
February 12, 2003

carvedilol reduced death and total hospitalizations by 19% to 49% when added to standard treatment for heart failure. There is also some interest in whether the amino acid L-arginine may improve blood flow in patients with heart failure.

A new drug option for people with heart failure is eplerenone (Inspra), which blocks the activity of the hormone aldosterone. It was approved by the FDA in October 2003. A recent study found that eplerenone improved survival in people who developed heart failure after a heart attack (see the sidebar at right).

Intravenous drugs are sometimes used when patients are admitted to the hospital because of worsening heart failure. These drugs include milrinone (Primacor), dobutamine (Dobutrex), nitroprusside (Nitropress), nitroglycerin (Nitro-Bid I.V., Tridil), and nesiritide (Natrecor).

People with class IV heart failure may require a heart transplant if other treatments prove ineffective. Donor hearts are in short supply, however, and individuals may have to wait a long time before one becomes available. During this period, a mechanical pump called a left ventricular assist device (LVAD) can help the heart work more effectively. LVADs also may spur significant recovery in hearts thought to be irreversibly damaged. In several cases, heart function improved so much that the patients were eventually weaned from the LVAD and no longer required a heart transplant. There is also hope that LVADs might serve as a permanent assist device for failing hearts and eliminate the need for transplants in some patients.

In 2001, the FDA approved the InSync cardiac pacing system, the first pacemaker for treating the symptoms of moderate to severe heart failure. This special pacemaker is intended for heart failure patients who have not responded adequately to medication and have a heart rhythm disturbance in which the two ventricles do not contract at the same time. The pacing system consists of a small pulse generator, implanted under the skin in the upper part of the chest near the shoulder, as well as insulated wires that deliver electrical signals from the generator to the heart's ventricles to stimulate them to contract simultaneously.

A clinical trial of InSync showed that more than two thirds of people using the device experienced improved symptoms, as demonstrated by an improvement in their heart failure class, while only one third of placebo patients did so. The device also improved quality of life, increased the distance patients could walk, and decreased the number of days spent in the hospital because of heart failure. People

NEW RESEARCH

New Drug for Heart Failure After Heart Attack

Eplerenone (Inspra), a newly approved medication, can help prevent deaths in people who have heart failure and left ventricular dysfunction after a heart attack, researchers report.

The study randomized 6,632 people with a recent heart attack complicated by heart failure and left ventricular dysfunction to receive either eplerenone (25 to 50 mg per day) or a placebo, in addition to their regular medical therapy. Over 16 months, the patients who took eplerenone were 15% to 21% less likely to die of cardiovascular disease, sudden cardiac death, or any cause than patients taking the placebo. Hospitalizations for cardiovascular events, such as heart failure, were similarly reduced in the eplerenone group.

Blood pressure increased during the study in both groups, but it increased less in the eplerenone group. Seriously elevated blood potassium levels occurred more frequently in patients taking eplerenone.

The authors conclude that eplerenone may reduce deaths and cardiovascular events in some patients following a heart attack and that one life could be saved per year for every 50 eligible people treated with eplerenone in addition to other optimal therapy.

THE NEW ENGLAND JOURNAL OF MEDICINE
Volume 348, page 1309
April 3, 2003

Drugs for Heart Failure 2004

Drug Type	Generic Name	Brand Name	Average Daily Dosage*	Wholesale Cost (Generic Cost)†
Loop diuretics	bumetanide	Bumex	0.5 to 2 mg	0.5 mg: $40 ($30)
	furosemide	Lasix	20 to 80 mg	40 mg: $34 ($14)
Thiazide diuretics	bendroflumethiazide	Naturetin-5	2.5 to 20 mg	5 mg: $119
	chlorothiazide	Diuril	250 to 1000 mg	250 mg: $17 ($12)
	chlorthalidone	Thalitone	25 to 100 mg	15 mg: $97 (25 mg: $14)
	hydrochlorothiazide/ triamterene	Dyazide	25 to 75 mg	25 mg/37.5 mg: $52 ($19)
	hydrochlorothiazide	Ezide	25 to 100 mg	50 mg: $4 (25 mg: $7)
		HydroDIURIL	25 to 100 mg	25 mg: $17 ($17)
	indapamide	Lozol	1.5 to 5 mg	2.5 mg: $119 ($79)
	methyclothiazide	Enduron	2.5 to 5 mg	5 mg: $77 ($52)
	metolazone	Zaroxolyn	2.5 to 5 mg	5 mg: $124
	trichlormethiazide	Naqua	2 to 4 mg	4 mg: $85 ($10)
Potassium-sparing diuretic	spironolactone	Aldactone	25 to 50 mg	25 mg: $65 ($46)
ACE inhibitors	captopril	Capoten	100 to 300 mg	12.5 mg: $119 ($69)
	enalapril	Vasotec	5 to 40 mg	10 mg: $125 ($105)
	lisinopril	Prinivil	2.5 to 20 mg	10 mg: $107 (5 mg: $45)
		Zestril	2.5 to 20 mg	10 mg: $115 (5 mg: $45)
	ramipril	Altace	10 mg	10 mg: $169
Beta-blockers	carvedilol	Coreg	12.5 mg	12.5 mg: $173
	metoprolol	Lopressor	100 to 400 mg	100 mg: $137 ($76)
	metoprolol, extended-release	Toprol XL	up to 400 mg	100 mg: $114
Cardiac glycosides	digoxin	Lanoxin	0.05 to 0.35 mg	0.125 mg: $23 ($15)
Aldosterone blockers	eplerenone	Inspra	25 to 50 mg	n/a

* These dosages represent an average range for the treatment of heart failure. The precise effective dosage varies from patient to patient and depends on many factors. Do not make any changes in your medication without consulting your doctor.

† Average wholesale prices to pharmacists for 100 tablets or capsules of the dosage strength listed. Costs to consumers are higher. If a generic is available, the cost is listed in parentheses. Source: *Red Book, 2003* (Medical Economics Data, publishers).

using the InSync pacemaker should avoid strong sources of magnetic, radiation, and electrical energy, which may disrupt its functioning.

Arrhythmias

In many individuals, arrhythmias can be treated successfully with drugs, though these medications can have serious side effects. Some types of arrhythmias require the administration of an electrical stimulus to the heart to return the heart to its normal rhythm—a technique called electrical cardioversion. An increasing

Uses	Side Effects	Special Considerations
To reduce sodium and water accumulation that leads to swelling and breathlessness in people with heart failure.	Loop diuretics can cause dehydration, potassium loss, and changes in the acidity of the blood. Thiazide diuretics may cause potassium loss, elevated triglyceride and glucose (sugar) levels, decreased HDL cholesterol, gout, weakness, erectile dysfunction, and dizziness on standing. Potassium-sparing diuretics can raise potassium levels, a danger for people with kidney disease.	Usually used in conjunction with an ACE inhibitor and a beta-blocker.
To treat heart failure, high blood pressure, and left ventricular systolic dysfunction.	Impaired kidney function, cough, and abdominal pain.	Improvement in symptoms may take several weeks or months.
To treat class II or III heart failure after patients are stabilized on diuretics and ACE inhibitors.	Shortness of breath; pain or tightness in chest; swelling of ankles, feet, and lower legs; and depression.	Improvement in symptoms may take two to three months.
To treat heart failure and arrhythmias.	Dizziness, shortness of breath, mental changes, and nausea.	For improvement of symptoms, digoxin should be used with a diuretic, an ACE inhibitor, and a beta-blocker.
To treat heart failure after a heart attack. Also approved to treat high blood pressure.	Dizziness, fatigue, flu-like symptoms, diarrhea, and cough. High blood potassium is a rare but serious side effect.	Improves survival in people who develop heart failure after a heart attack. Used in combination with standard heart failure medications.

number of arrhythmias can be treated with radiofrequency catheter ablation, which suppresses or destroys an abnormal electrical circuit within the heart. In some cases, an implanted electrical device—such as a pacemaker or cardioverter-defibrillator—is used instead of, or in addition to, drugs.

Drugs. Arrhythmias may be treated with a variety of drugs, most of which suppress abnormal pacemaker activity in the heart or block conduction of abnormal electrical impulses.

In people with atrial fibrillation, aspirin or warfarin is generally prescribed to reduce the risk of blood clots in the heart. These blood clots are dangerous because they can travel through the bloodstream and become lodged in an artery supplying blood to the brain, causing a stroke.

Digoxin is frequently used to treat atrial fibrillation. By slowing the conduction of electrical impulses through the AV node, digoxin reduces the response of the ventricles to the rapid rhythm of the atria. Beta-blockers and calcium channel blockers also inhibit conduction through the AV node. Another useful drug is ibutilide (Corvert), which can quickly return the heart to its normal rhythm. Antiarrhythmic drugs such as procainamide (Pronestyl and other brands), sotalol (Betapace), amiodarone (Cordarone), flecainide (Tambocor), and propafenone (Rythmol) may also be used to control atrial fibrillation. These antiarrhythmic drugs have potentially serious side effects (for example, bradycardia and hypothyroidism).

The most effective drug for controlling ventricular arrhythmias varies from patient to patient. Electrophysiology studies (see pages 27–28) are often used to determine which drug is most likely to work best. Drugs that suppress ventricular arrhythmias through direct action on the ventricles include tocainide (Tonocard) and mexiletine (Mexitil). Other drugs that can help control ventricular arrhythmias include procainamide, sotalol, amiodarone, flecainide, and propafenone.

Electrical cardioversion. When drug therapy fails, electrical cardioversion may be tried for some arrhythmias to return the heart rhythm to normal. This approach is most commonly used for atrial fibrillation. After a sedative is administered intravenously, the heart is given an electrical shock using an external defibrillator. The electrical shock interrupts the heart's electrical activity and may help reinitiate a normal rhythm.

Emergency electrical cardioversion is the only effective treatment for ventricular fibrillation, which results in cardiac arrest, loss of consciousness, and death if not corrected within a few minutes. With the availability of portable external defibrillators, life-saving electrical cardioversion can be delivered by emergency personnel, the general public, or a family member. These defibrillators are available in ambulances and in public places such as shopping malls and sports arenas. A defibrillator for use at home was recently approved by the FDA (see the feature on pages 72–73).

Artificial pacemakers. Artificial pacemakers are surgically implanted devices that provide electrical stimuli to control heart rate in people whose heart rate is too slow or too fast. Implantation of

NEW RESEARCH

Implantable Device Effective for People With Heart Failure

A new implantable device appears to be beneficial for people with moderate to severe heart failure. The device combines an implantable cardioverter-defibrillator (ICD), to stop life-threatening ventricular arrhythmias, and cardiac resynchronization therapy (CRT), to help the heart beat in a more coordinated fashion.

Investigators studied 369 people with moderate to severe heart failure who were at high risk for life-threatening ventricular arrhythmias and were receiving standard medication. Half were randomly assigned to receive a device with both an active ICD and CRT while the other half received a device with an active ICD but an inactive CRT.

Six months later, those receiving both the active ICD and CRT were more likely to have improved quality of life, New York Heart Association functional class, and exercise ability than the group with the inactive CRT. The active ICD and CRT group also could exercise longer than the inactive CRT group. However, both groups could walk the same distance in six minutes.

An accompanying editorial points out that the combined ICD and CRT device is likely appropriate for only 5% of heart failure patients and that its effect on survival and any long-term complications still need to be determined.

JOURNAL OF THE AMERICAN MEDICAL ASSOCIATION
Volume 289, pages 2685 and 2719
May 28, 2003

the pacemaker is a minor surgical procedure performed under local anesthesia. First, two wires called leads are inserted into the heart through a vein in the neck. Then the pacemaker unit, which is slightly larger than a man's wristwatch, is placed just under the skin in the upper chest and attached to the leads. Most people are hospitalized overnight for observation after the procedure and can resume their normal schedule within two weeks.

The pacemaker must be tested periodically. Replacement of the unit, usually every 8 to 10 years, requires a minor operation.

Implantable cardioverter-defibrillators. An implantable cardioverter-defibrillator (ICD) can stop a life-threatening ventricular arrhythmia. It is used in people who have survived a cardiac arrest due to ventricular tachycardia or ventricular fibrillation and in people who are at high risk for these ventricular arrhythmias (for example, because they have had a heart attack with resulting left ventricular dysfunction).

When the device senses a rapid ventricular rate due to ventricular tachycardia or ventricular fibrillation, it automatically delivers an electrical shock to the heart to try to terminate the abnormal rhythm. The shock is very powerful; some people say it feels like being kicked in the chest. After receiving a shock, patients should contact their physician or go to a hospital for evaluation. Some ICD models can serve as a pacemaker as well.

Implantation of the ICD generally requires a two- to three-day hospital stay and a week-long recovery period at home. Most ICDs are implanted much like a pacemaker: One or two leads are inserted into the heart, and the device is placed under the skin in the chest or abdomen. Regular follow-up visits to the doctor are needed, and minor surgery is necessary every three to seven years to replace the unit.

Wearable defibrillator. A wearable defibrillator is an option for people who are temporarily at high risk for cardiac arrest, for example, those who are recovering from a heart attack or waiting for a heart transplant. The defibrillator, approved in 2001, is a vest-like device that is worn under clothing. An electrode in the vest is able to detect abnormal, life-threatening heart rhythms and deliver an electrical shock to restore the heart's rhythm to normal. To learn more about the wearable defibrillator, see the feature on pages 72–73.

Radiofrequency catheter ablation. Radiofrequency catheter ablation is an increasingly popular method to suppress arrhythmias such as ventricular tachycardia. It involves an electrophysiology study to

NEW RESEARCH

Airport Metal Detectors Likely Do Not Affect Heart Devices

People with heart devices such as pacemakers and implantable cardioverter defibrillators (ICDs) can safely pass through airport metal detectors, a new study finds. People with these devices carry medical cards and currently are not required to walk through the metal detectors. The researchers undertook the study because many patients were concerned that recent increases in airport security measures would require them to pass through the detectors anyway.

The researchers sent 348 people with heart devices through a type of metal detector used at most airports in the United States, Canada, and Europe. The sensitivity of the pacemakers was not adjusted before the test, but the ICDs were set to the highest sensitivity (although the part of the device that delivers a shock was turned off). Participants walked back and forth through the metal detector at a normal walking pace. They also stood in the metal detector for at least 20 seconds and then turned so that their chests faced the sensors.

During the test, none of the participants had heart rhythm abnormalities on an electrocardiogram (ECG), and none of the devices delivered unnecessary therapies or underwent spontaneous reprogramming.

JOURNAL OF THE AMERICAN COLLEGE OF CARDIOLOGY
Volume 41, page 2054
June 4, 2003

External Defibrillators

New devices that can be worn or kept at home help people receive treatment more quickly for life-threatening heart arrhythmias.

Each year, up to 250,000 people in the United States die of cardiac arrest. Cardiac arrest is usually caused by an arrhythmia called ventricular fibrillation, in which the ventricles quiver chaotically and the heart is unable to pump blood to the rest of the body. Cardiopulmonary resuscitation (CPR) can keep blood flowing to the brain, but the arrhythmia can only be corrected with a defibrillator, which sends an electrical shock into the heart to try to re-establish a normal rhythm.

Cardiac arrest is most likely in men over the age of 45, and factors like an unhealthy lifestyle, symptoms of coronary heart disease, or a family history of heart disease can increase the risk. However, many people who die of cardiac arrest have no prior symptoms of heart disease.

If a person experiences a cardiac arrest (usually indicated by a collapse and loss of consciousness, along with lack of a heartbeat), someone nearby should call 911 immediately.

The current survival rate for cardiac arrest in the United States is less than 5%, because emergency personnel often cannot reach the person in time. Although defibrillation is effective, it must be delivered within a few minutes of the loss of heartbeat. People defibrillated within five minutes have a 50% survival rate; for each minute that passes without CPR or defibrillation, a person in cardiac arrest is 7% to 10% less likely to survive. In a typical community, it takes an ambulance nine minutes to reach someone in cardiac arrest.

Most people are familiar with the external defibrillators that are used in hospitals for people with ventricular fibrillation. In the mid-1990s, the American Heart Association began to promote the use of modified versions (called automated external defibrillators, or AEDs) in places where large groups of people gather, in the hope of providing treatment more quickly.

Because AEDs are relatively simple to operate, they are becoming more widely available in public areas (such as shopping malls and sports arenas), as well as in places (such as airplanes or cruise ships) that are not accessible to emergency personnel. These devices analyze the heart rhythm and automatically administer a shock if it is necessary. Some training is required to learn how to evaluate patients properly and to use the device correctly.

The American Heart Association estimates that more than 40,000 deaths could be prevented each year if defibrillators were more widely available in public places. In addition, external defibrillators that can be worn on the body or kept in the home have recently received U.S. Food and Drug Administration (FDA) approval. They may benefit people at increased risk for cardiac arrest.

Home Defibrillators

Some people at risk for cardiac arrest keep a regular AED in their homes. However, in November 2002, the FDA approved the first AED designed specifically for the home. The device is easier to use and less expensive than the type used in public places.

Home AEDs may be valuable for treating cardiac arrest because more than 70% of these events happen in the home, and most are witnessed by a family member or other person who could provide help. The home AED may particularly benefit adults who need an implantable defibrillator but are too old or ill to undergo the surgical procedure to implant it.

The voice coaching on the home defibrillator is more comprehensive than that used in other AEDs, and it is

detect the area of the heart responsible for generating the abnormal rhythm. The area is then destroyed using radiofrequency energy delivered through a catheter. The effectiveness of this outpatient technique is high in appropriate patients, and the risk is minimal.

HEART TRANSPLANTATION

A heart transplant is considered when heart failure produces severe symptoms and life expectancy is greatly limited. Transplant recipients should be younger than age 60 and have no other major diseases simple enough for even a sixth-grade child to understand. The voice commands, which are automatically adjusted to match the speed of the user's actions, remind the relative or other bystander to call for emergency help and tell the user to attach the pads to the patient's chest. The device assesses the heart rhythm and eliminates the risk of an unnecessary shock by determining whether defibrillation is required.

The home defibrillator also guides the user through the steps of CPR. When not in use, the device performs daily self-tests and chirps when it needs maintenance, much like a smoke alarm does when it needs new batteries.

Some experts have expressed concern that distraught relatives and friends may waste precious time during an emergency looking for the home defibrillator or discovering that the batteries are dead, instead of calling 911 immediately. Some also worry that people with heart disease may rely on the defibrillator, instead of taking their medication and making diet and exercise changes.

The National Institutes of Health has begun a study of 7,000 people at high risk for cardiac arrest to see how well family members are able to use an at-home defibrillator in an emergency. Until the device is shown to save lives, the American Heart Association does not recommend its use.

The home defibrillator, which costs about $2,000, requires a doctor's prescription. It is not yet clear whether Medicare or other insurance companies will reimburse patients. Although the defibrillator is easy to use and comes with an owner's manual and instructional video, the American Heart Association recommends that potential users complete training in CPR and AEDs. This training will help relatives and friends recognize the signs of cardiac arrest and become familiar with the device, both of which can save time in a life-threatening situation. To find a training center, call 877-AHA-4CPR or visit the American Heart Association's Web site (www.americanheart.org/ cpr). (For more information on the home defibrillator, call 866-333-4246 or visit www.heartstarthome.com.)

Wearable Defibrillators

A defibrillator that can be worn outside the body was approved by the FDA in 2001 for some people who are recovering from a heart attack or are waiting for a heart transplant. Such people are temporarily at high risk for cardiac arrest. The device is designed to perform like an implantable defibrillator but without the expense and risks of surgery.

The wearable defibrillator consists of a fabric holster that is worn over the shoulders and strapped to the chest with an alarm module at the waist. Sensors automatically monitor the patient's heartbeat 24 hours a day. If the sensors detect an abnormal rhythm, an alarm alerts the wearer to press two buttons on the alarm module. The device delivers a shock only if the patient loses consciousness and is unable to press the buttons. This approach prevents the device from shocking the wearer while conscious, which can be painful.

The device is meant to be worn continuously, although patients should remove it to shower or bathe. The battery needs to be charged every 24 hours.

Studies of the wearable defibrillator in 289 patients found that it successfully treated cardiac arrest in 71% of cases, compared with 25% of people who call 911 and wait for help to arrive. The device delivered inappropriate shocks to 2% of the users, which is similar to the rate in people with implantable defibrillators. The most common side effect of wearing the defibrillator is a temporary skin rash, which is experienced by 5% of people.

Because the device is meant to be used only for short periods, it is available for rental instead of purchase. Medicare and most insurance companies cover the cost of renting the device. (For more information about the wearable defibrillator, call 800-LIFECOR or visit www.lifecor.com.)

like cancer or kidney disease that might shorten their life span.

The success of heart transplants has improved markedly over the past decade: About 84% of transplant patients are alive after one year, and 71% survive for at least five years. These improvements in survival are primarily the result of advances in the prevention and early diagnosis of rejection, in which the immune system recognizes the donated heart as foreign and attempts to destroy it.

Medications must be taken to suppress the immune system, and regular biopsies of the heart are needed to identify early rejection. The medications routinely used to suppress the immune system include cyclosporine (Neoral, Sandimmune), azathioprine (Imuran), and prednisone (Deltasone and other brands). The biopsies are performed under local anesthesia and involve inserting a small tube into a vein and advancing the tube to the heart. A small piece of tissue is then removed from the heart and examined under the microscope.

Many people with a transplanted heart develop CHD in their new heart. The risk of CHD may be reduced, in part, by the same lifestyle changes and medications used to prevent CHD in nontransplant patients. In addition, calcium channel blockers and statins seem to slow the development of CHD. To monitor for CHD, heart transplant patients should undergo coronary angiography once a year.

ARTIFICIAL HEART IMPLANTATION

In July 2001, the FDA gave permission for researchers to test an artificial heart in 15 patients. Called the AbioCor Implantable Replacement Heart, it weighs 2 lbs., is surgically implanted in the chest, and is powered by electricity that passes though intact skin from an external battery.

The artificial heart is designed for people with end-stage heart failure who are unable to undergo a transplant. The results so far indicate that many of the artificial heart recipients live longer than they would have without the device, but complications are numerous and include serious bleeding, blood clots, strokes, and lung infections. Even if subsequent investigations show the device is successful, it may be years before the artificial heart comes into regular use.

CARDIAC REHABILITATION

Doctors have learned the importance of rehabilitation after a heart attack. For years, the popular belief was that a heart attack signaled the end of an active, healthy life. Today, however, better knowledge of how the heart works has made cardiac rehabilitation the cornerstone of recovery after a heart attack (as well as after bypass surgery or angioplasty). Indeed, many people who follow a prescribed rehabilitation plan are healthier and more active than they were before the heart attack.

In-Hospital Rehabilitation

Typically, rehabilitation begins while patients are still in the hospital. Since too much bed rest may cause weakness and prolong the time and effort of recovery, patients are encouraged to begin moving around within one to two days of a heart attack.

Activity is resumed slowly in a series of progressive steps: sitting up in bed; sitting in a chair; performing simple range-of-motion exercises; and, finally, taking short walks around the room or down the hall. During these activities, the patients' heart rhythms are closely monitored. Most heart attack patients are ready to leave the hospital within five to seven days, but a longer stay may be needed for those with complications such as arrhythmias, heart failure, or recurrent chest pain.

Before leaving the hospital, paticnts usually are given an exercise stress test to measure the heart's electrical activity during modest physical exertion. Based on these results, doctors can prescribe an individualized exercise plan for the patient to follow over the next several weeks. At this time, the doctor also will recommend an appropriate outpatient rehabilitation program. In certain cases, rehabilitation at home may be recommended instead.

Patient education also should begin in the hospital and continue in the outpatient rehabilitation program. Individual consultations or group sessions on improving diet and quitting smoking, for example, should start before a patient leaves the hospital. In addition, the emotional stress of having a heart attack often requires immediate psychological counseling, as patients grapple with such issues as fear of dying or having another heart attack and anxiety about returning to their job or resuming sexual activity. Counseling also should continue during outpatient rehabilitation as needed.

Outpatient Rehabilitation

The primary goals of outpatient cardiac rehabilitation programs are to maximize physical strength and endurance; minimize the occurrence of ischemia, angina, and future heart attacks; alleviate anxiety about resuming physical activity; aid in weight control; ease patients back into their daily routines; and improve their quality of life and understanding of their condition.

The main component of all rehabilitation programs is supervised exercise. In general, the goal is to gradually work up to a standard aerobic workout—5 to 10 minutes of warm-up and stretching, 20 to 40 minutes of aerobic activity (such as walking, jogging, or swimming), and 5 minutes of cool-down and stretching—at least three times a week. The pace and type of workout are tailored to the individual, taking into consideration the condition of the heart, as well as any other illnesses. Light weight training also may be included.

The best rehabilitation programs also offer comprehensive, personalized advice and support on dietary measures, smoking cessation, and stress control, as well as psychosocial services for such issues as anxiety, depression, and family or occupational problems. The emphasis should be on long-term maintenance of a healthy lifestyle. In addition, all cardiac rehabilitation sites should have emergency cardiac equipment and medical personnel available.

The major advantage of a structured outpatient rehabilitation program is the continual encouragement to improve lifestyle habits. In addition, most people find it helpful to share their experiences with other heart attack survivors. If possible, patients should stick with the outpatient program for at least two months to increase the chances of retaining new habits over the long term. Some programs offer a maintenance phase (usually 6 to 12 months) that continues even after patients have recuperated enough to return to work and other normal activities.

DEPRESSION

Depression is common in people with CHD: While 5% of Americans suffer from depression in a given year, about 20% of people with CHD are depressed.

Depression in people with CHD is associated with more severe disease and a higher risk of death, particularly in those recovering from a heart attack. For example, depressed heart attack patients are more likely to have a subsequent CHD event (such as another heart attack) and are more likely to die within 18 months than heart attack patients who are not depressed. Recent studies also suggest that depression is a risk factor for CHD events in people with unstable angina or heart failure.

It is unclear how depression leads to poor outcomes in people with CHD, but researchers have proposed two possible explanations. First, depression can result in a rapid heart rate, high blood pressure, arrhythmias, faster blood clotting, and elevated blood levels of insulin and cholesterol—all of which can lead to a worse outcome. Second, people with both depression and CHD are less likely to take their medications regularly, participate in a cardiac rehabilitation program, or make recommended lifestyle changes (such as exercising, eating a low-fat diet, and quitting smoking).

Fortunately, depression is a treatable condition. Treatment options include antidepressant drugs, psychotherapy, or a combination of both. Studies show that psychotherapy alleviates depression

NEW RESEARCH

Antidepressant May Lower Risk of Blood Clotting

Depression increases the risk of heart attack and stroke, possibly by activating platelets, which are cells involved in blood clotting. Now, researchers have shown that treatment of depression in heart patients using a type of antidepressant known as a selective serotonin reuptake inhibitor (SSRI) can decrease platelet activation.

The study involved 64 people who were hospitalized for either a heart attack or unstable angina and also had major depression. They were randomized to receive either the SSRI sertraline (Zoloft) or a placebo; they were also prescribed medications for their heart condition, including anticoagulants, aspirin, and other antiplatelet drugs.

The researchers performed eight different tests of platelet activation. After 16 weeks, platelet activation was significantly decreased for seven of eight tests in patients assigned to sertraline, compared with only five of eight tests for those assigned to the placebo.

A decreased capacity for blood clotting may partly explain why treatment of depression in heart attack patients tends to improve survival. The authors suggest that the benefits of SSRIs might extend to heart patients who are not depressed. They also note that up to a quarter of people who experience a heart attack develop major depression.

CIRCULATION
Volume 108, page 939
August 26, 2003

in people with CHD and helps them make necessary lifestyle changes. Early results also suggest that antidepressants such as selective serotonin reuptake inhibitors (SSRIs) and bupropion (Wellbutrin) are safe and effective in people with CHD. For example, in a recent study of more than 350 people with unstable angina or a recent heart attack, the SSRI sertraline (Zoloft) effectively reduced symptoms of depression without having a negative effect on the heart. Tricyclic antidepressants are used less often because they can cause dangerous arrhythmias in people with heart disease. Social support and exercise also can improve depression in people with CHD. ■

GLOSSARY

aneurysm—A ballooning of the wall of the heart, an artery, or a vein caused by weakening of the wall.

angina—An episode of pain, pressure, or tightness in the chest caused by an imbalance between the supply of oxygen to the heart muscle and the heart muscle's need for oxygen. Angina occurs most often during increased physical activity or emotional stress. Also called angina pectoris.

angiography—The best method of detecting blockages within the coronary arteries and determining the severity of the blockages. Contrast material is injected through a catheter into the coronary arteries while x-rays are taken of the arteries.

angioplasty—In this procedure, a catheter with a balloon at its tip is directed to a site where a coronary artery is narrowed by plaque. The balloon is inflated to decrease the size of the plaque and stretch the artery. Also called percutaneous transluminal coronary angioplasty (PTCA).

anticoagulants—Drugs that decrease the formation of blood clots by inhibiting the production of fibrin, a protein required for clots to form. Examples are heparin and warfarin (Coumadin).

antioxidants—Substances that help the body neutralize free radicals. Beta-carotene, vitamin E, and vitamin C are naturally occurring antioxidants.

antiplatelets—Drug that decrease the formation of blood clots by inhibiting the aggregation or clumping of blood cells called platelets. One example is aspirin.

aorta—The body's main artery. It transports oxygenated blood from the left ventricle of the heart to the arteries that supply the rest of the body.

arrhythmia—An abnormal heart rhythm.

atherectomy—A method of removing plaque from the inside of an artery using a rotary blade or drill.

atherosclerosis—An accumulation of deposits of fat and fibrous tissue, called plaques, within the walls of arteries that can narrow the arteries and reduce blood flow through them.

atria—The two upper chambers of the heart. The left atrium receives newly oxygenated blood from the lungs; the right atrium receives deoxygenated blood returning from the rest of the body.

atrial fibrillation—A common heart rhythm abnormality in which the atria contract at a rapid, chaotic rate and cause rapid and irregular pumping of the ventricles.

body mass index (BMI)—A measurement of weight in relation to height. Calculated by multiplying weight in pounds by 704 and dividing the result by the square of height in inches. Overweight is defined as a BMI of 25 to 29.9 and obesity as a BMI of 30 and over.

bradycardia—A heart rhythm characterized by a slow heart rate. Usually defined as less than 45 beats per minute in an adult.

bypass surgery—A surgical procedure in which an artery from the chest or a portion of a vein from the leg is used to channel blood around a narrowed segment of a coronary artery. Also called coronary artery bypass graft surgery (CABG).

cardiac arrest—A sudden, abrupt loss of the heart's ability to pump blood, most often as a result of ventricular fibrillation.

cardiac catheterization—A procedure in which a thin plastic tube is introduced through an artery in the arm or leg. From there, the tube is advanced into the coronary arteries or heart for diagnostic or therapeutic purposes.

cardiac output—The amount of blood pumped by the heart.

cardiovascular disease—Disease affecting the heart or arterial vascular system of the body. Coronary heart disease, stroke, and peripheral vascular disease are the most common cardiovascular diseases.

cerebrovascular disease—Disease that affects arteries supplying blood to the brain.

cholesterol—A soft, waxy substance present in cells throughout the body. Deposition of cholesterol within the walls of arteries can lead to the formation of atherosclerotic plaques.

congestive heart failure—See **heart failure**.

coronary artery bypass graft surgery (CABG)—See **bypass surgery**.

coronary artery disease—See **coronary heart disease**.

coronary event—See **coronary heart disease event**.

coronary heart disease (CHD)—A narrowing of the coronary arteries by atherosclerosis. Can reduce or completely block blood flow to the heart. Also called coronary artery disease.

coronary heart disease (CHD) event—Often defined as a heart attack, episode of unstable angina, or CHD-related death. Also called a coronary event.

defibrillation—Use of an electric shock to reestablish a normal rhythm in a heart that is beating ineffectively due to ventricular fibrillation.

diastolic blood pressure—The lower number in a blood pressure reading. The pressure in the arteries when the heart relaxes between beats.

echocardiography—A diagnostic test that uses ultrasound waves to visualize the heart, its valves, and the flow of blood within the heart.

ejection fraction—The percentage of the blood in the left ventricle that is pumped from the heart with each contraction. The ejection fraction ranges from 50% to 65% in a healthy person.

electrocardiogram (ECG or EKG)—A graphical record of the heart's electrical activity obtained by applying small metal sensors to the skin. Used to detect abnormal heart rhythms and heart damage.

embolus—A blood clot or piece of atherosclerotic plaque that breaks loose and travels through the bloodstream. It can block blood flow by lodging in an artery. The plural form is emboli.

endothelium—The layer of cells that line the walls of arteries. Injury to these cells is an important first step in the development of atherosclerosis.

free radicals—Chemical compounds formed during normal metabolism. They can damage cells and oxidize low density lipoproteins, which can then be deposited in the walls of arteries.

heart attack—Tissue death caused by insufficient blood supply to a portion of the heart muscle. Technically known as myocardial infarction.

heart failure—A condition in which the heart is unable to pump enough blood to meet the needs of the body. Common signs of heart failure include shortness of breath and accumulation of fluid in the lungs, legs, and abdomen.

high density lipoprotein (HDL)—A protein that protects against atherosclerosis by removing cholesterol deposited in artery walls.

Holter monitor—A portable device worn to monitor the heart's rhythm over an extended time, often 24 hours. Also called an ambulatory electrocardiogram.

homocysteine—An amino acid required for normal body function. High levels in the blood may promote atherosclerosis by damaging the endothelium and stimulating formation of blood clots.

hormone replacement therapy (HRT)—A combination of estrogen and progestin (a synthetic form of progesterone) used by women to relieve the symptoms of menopause and reduce bone loss. Not recommended for the prevention of CHD or CHD events.

hypertension—High blood pressure.

ischemia—An inadequate supply of blood to any part of the body. Ischemia to the heart muscle may cause chest pain.

laser ablation—A method of removing plaque from the inside of an artery using heat from a laser.

lipoprotein—A protein that transports cholesterol and other fats in the blood.

lipoprotein(a)— A lipoprotein with a structure similar to low density lipoprotein but containing another protein called apo(a). High levels of lipoprotein(a) are a risk factor for coronary heart disease. Also called Lp(a).

low density lipoprotein (LDL)—A protein that transports cholesterol in the bloodstream. A major contributor to atherosclerosis.

monounsaturated fat—A type of fat found in avocados, almonds, and olive and canola oils. Can lower LDL cholesterol levels and stabilize or raise HDL cholesterol levels when substituted for saturated fat in the diet.

myocardial infarction—See **heart attack**.

myocardium—The muscle of the heart.

pacemaker—An implanted, battery-operated device that can take the place of the heart's normal pacemaker when an abnormality in pacemaker function occurs.

percutaneous transluminal coronary angioplasty—See **angioplasty**.

peripheral vascular disease—A narrowing of the arteries in the extremities, usually the legs. Commonly due to atherosclerosis.

plaque—An accumulation of cholesterol-laden foam cells, smooth muscle cells, fibrous proteins, and calcium in the wall of an artery.

polyunsaturated fat—A type of fat found in safflower, sunflower, and corn oils. Can lower LDL cholesterol when substituted for saturated fat in the diet.

radiofrequency catheter ablation—A technique for treating arrhythmias that uses radio waves to suppress or destroy an abnormal electrical circuit within the heart.

restenosis—Narrowing of an artery after angioplasty.

revascularization—A procedure to improve blood supply to the heart. Usually refers to bypass surgery or angioplasty.

saturated fat—A type of fat that includes most animal fats and some oils, such as palm and coconut oils. A major dietary factor in raising blood cholesterol.

stable angina—Angina triggered by a predictable amount of activity or stress. The characteristics of the pain are similar in each attack, and the pain is usually relieved by rest or a nitrate drug. It is the most common type of angina.

stent—A wire mesh tube that is permanently inserted into a coronary artery during angioplasty to help keep it open.

GLOSSARY—continued

systolic blood pressure—The upper number in a blood pressure reading. The pressure in the arteries when the heart is pumping blood.

tachycardia—A heart rhythm abnormality characterized by a heart rate higher than 100 beats per minute at rest.

trans fatty acids—Fats formed when food manufacturers add hydrogen atoms to unsaturated fats to make them more saturated and therefore more solid and shelf-stable. Found in margarines and store-bought baked goods. Trans fatty acids raise blood cholesterol.

triglyceride—A lipid (fat) that is a storage form of energy. High levels of triglycerides in the blood contribute to atherosclerosis.

unstable angina—A condition intermediate in severity between stable angina and a heart attack. Caused by a blood clot or spasm in a coronary artery. Sometimes called crescendo angina.

ventricles—The two chambers in the lower part of the heart. The left ventricle receives oxygenated blood from the left atrium and pumps it to the rest of the body; the right ventricle receives deoxygenated blood from the right atrium and pumps it to the lungs.

ventricular fibrillation—A heart rhythm abnormality in which the pumping action of the ventricles is completely lost. Death occurs within a few minutes unless resuscitation is successful.

ventricular tachycardia—A heart rhythm abnormality that originates in the ventricles and produces a heart rate faster than 100 beats per minute.

very low density lipoprotein (VLDL)—A protein that is the major carrier of triglycerides in the bloodstream.

HEALTH INFORMATION ORGANIZATIONS AND SUPPORT GROUPS

American College of Cardiology
9111 Old Georgetown Rd.
Bethesda, MD 20814-1699
☎ 800-253-4636/301-897-5400
www.acc.org

Professional medical society and teaching institution that provides professional education, promotes research, offers leadership in the development of standards and guidelines, and forms health care policy.

American Dietetic Association
120 S. Riverside Plaza, Ste. 2000
Chicago, IL 60606-6995
☎ 800-366-1655/312-899-0040
www.eatright.org

Provides recorded nutrition messages, helps consumers locate registered dietitians for counseling, and provides answers to food and nutrition questions related to heart-healthy eating.

American Heart Association
7272 Greenville Ave.
Dallas, TX 75231
☎ 800-242-8721
www.americanheart.org

National health organization that provides information and public education programs on all aspects of heart disease. Check for local chapters.

Mended Hearts, Inc.
7272 Greenville Ave.
Dallas, TX 75231-4596
☎ 888-HEART-99/214-706-1442
www.mendedhearts.org

Support group for heart disease patients and their families. Call, write, or visit the Web site for information and to get in touch with other heart patients in your area.

National Heart, Lung, and Blood Institute Information Center
P.O. Box 30105
Bethesda, MD 20824-0105
☎ 800-575-WELL/301-592-8573
www.nhlbi.nih.gov/health/infoctr/index.htm

Branch of the National Institutes of Health that provides written information on all heart-related issues.

National Rehabilitation Information Center
4200 Forbes Blvd., Ste. 202
Lanham, MD 20706
☎ 800-346-2742/301-459-5900
301-459-5984 (TTY)
www.naric.com

Information center with database of literature and information on thousands of products and devices devoted to rehabilitation, including cardiac rehabilitation.

LEADING HOSPITALS FOR CARDIOLOGY AND HEART SURGERY

U.S. News & World Report and the National Opinion Research Center, a social-science research group at the University of Chicago, recently conducted their 14th annual nationwide survey of 8,160 physicians in 17 medical specialties. The doctors nominated up to five hospitals they consider best from among 6,003 U.S. hospitals. This is the current list of the best hospitals for cardiology and heart surgery, as determined by the doctors' recommendations from 2001, 2002, and 2003; federal data on death rates; and factual data regarding quality indicators, such as the ratio of registered nurses to patients and the use of advanced technology. Since the results reflect doctors' opinions, however, they are subjective to some degree. Any institution listed is considered a leading center, and the rankings do not imply that other hospitals cannot or do not deliver excellent care.

1. **Cleveland Clinic**
   Cleveland, OH
   ☎ 800-223-2273/216-444-2200
   www.clevelandclinic.org

2. **Mayo Clinic**
   Rochester, MN
   ☎ 507-284-2511
   www.mayoclinic.org

3. **Brigham and Women's Hospital**
   Boston, MA
   ☎ 617-732-5500
   www.brighamandwomens.org

4. **Duke University Medical Center**
   Durham, NC
   ☎ 919-684-8111
   www.mc.duke.edu

5. **Massachusetts General Hospital**
   Boston, MA
   ☎ 617-726-2000
   www.mgh.harvard.edu

6. **Johns Hopkins Hospital**
   Baltimore, MD
   ☎ 800-507-9952/410-955-5000
   www.hopkinsmedicine.org

7. **Emory University Hospital**
   Atlanta, GA
   ☎ 800-75-EMORY/404-778-7777
   www.emoryhealthcare.org

8. **Texas Heart Institute at St. Luke's Episcopal Hospital**
   Houston, TX
   ☎ 800-292-2221
   www.texasheartinstitute.org

9. **Stanford Hospital and Clinics**
   Stanford, CA
   ☎ 650-723-4000
   www.stanfordhospital.com

10. **Barnes-Jewish Hospital**
    St. Louis, MO
    ☎ 314-747-3000
    www.barnesjewish.org

RESTENOSIS: PREVENTING A COMMON COMPLICATION

A common problem after angioplasty is restenosis—a narrowing of the treated artery. Researchers have investigated numerous methods of preventing this complication and have made many advances in recent years. In a review, reprinted here from the *British Medical Journal,* Balram Bhargava, M.D., and colleagues discuss these new therapies.

Restenosis involves three separate processes. The first, vessel recoil, is the tendency of the artery wall to return to its constricted state after being stretched open by the angioplasty balloon. The second, neointimal proliferation, is the migration and proliferation of smooth muscle cells to the intima (the innermost lining of the injured artery). The third is thrombus formation, the accumulation of platelets and other factors to form a blood clot.

One way doctors have tried to combat restenosis is with oral drugs. This approach, which tries to prevent inflammation and blood clot formation, has met with limited success. Placing a stent in the treated artery can eliminate vessel recoil, but the artery is still at risk for neointimal proliferation and blood clot formation. As a result, doctors have now begun to use stents that are coated with drugs.

Stents coated with the drug heparin help prevent blood clot formation, but the drug is permanently bound to the stent and not released. Coated stents that release drugs over time to the nearby tissue are called drug-eluting stents. One of these stents, called the Cypher stent, elutes the antibiotic sirolimus and was recently approved by the U.S. Food and Drug Administration. (For more on this stent, see the feature on pages 60–61.) Another stent releases the drug paclitaxel, an anticancer drug. These and other drug-eluting stents, which help prevent neointimal proliferation, are associated with a "near zero percent" rate of restenosis, Dr. Bhargava and colleagues write. They optimistically call these drug-eluting stents the potential "final phase" in the evolution of techniques to prevent restenosis.

The authors also discuss other investigational methods for preventing restenosis, including biodegradable stents, debulking devices (which scrape away the plaque in the artery), gene and radiation therapy to control scarring, and cutting balloon angioplasty (in which the plaque is sliced, allowing it to be compressed more easily by angioplasty).

New approaches to preventing restenosis

Balram Bhargava, Ganesan Karthikeyan, Alexandre S Abizaid, Roxana Mehran

For over a quarter of a century percutaneous coronary interventions have been used to treat patients with coronary artery disease, yet restenosis continues to be a problem. This review discusses the advances being made to overcome restenosis, particularly the development of drug eluting stents

Department of Cardiology, Cardiothoracic Sciences Center, All India Institute of Medical Sciences, New Delhi 110029, India
Balram Bhargava *senior consultant*
Ganesan Karthikeyan *consultant*

Dante Pazzanese Institute of Cardiology, Sao Paulo, Brazil
Alexandre S Abizaid *consultant*

Cardiovascular Research Foundation, New York, NY, USA
Roxana Mehran *consultant*

Correspondence to: B Bhargava balrambhargava@yahoo.com

BMJ 2003;327:274–9

Additional web references (w1-w53) and tables appear on bmj.com

Andreas Gruntzig pioneered percutaneous transluminal coronary angioplasty in 1977.[1] Since then, percutaneous coronary interventions have revolutionised the treatment of patients with symptoms of coronary artery disease, sparing them the need for surgical revascularisation. In the United States, the number of percutaneous interventions performed each year is nearly double that of coronary artery bypass surgery.[w1] There have been three phases in the evolution of percutaneous interventions (see box 1), but in each restenosis has been a problem. It seems the next (and optimistically the final) phase is the development of drug eluting stents—that is, stents used for the local delivery of drugs (table).

Summary points

Restenosis is a common problem after percutaneous coronary interventions, depending on patient characteristics, lesion morphology, and the type of intervention

Coronary stenting is the only intervention that has reliably and consistently reduced restenosis in coronary lesions

Near zero per cent restenosis rates have recently been achieved with antiproliferative drug eluting coronary stents

Recurrent stenosis after treatment of instent restenosis is common

Adjuvant treatment with intracoronary γ and β radiation is the most effective currently available means to prevent recurrent stenosis after the treatment of instent restenosis

Modifying gene expression using antisense therapies or gene transfer will play an important part in the prevention of restenosis

Sources and selection criteria

The information in this review is based on the results of a Medline search using the key words coronary angioplasty, restenosis, instent restenosis, drug eluting stents, and intracoronary brachytherapy, and articles from the authors' personal collection. Cross references and related articles were accessed when necessary.

Restenosis

Restenosis is the maladaptive response of the coronary artery to injury. The simplest and most widely used definition of restenosis is a diameter stenosis of 50% at follow up. Restenosis occurs in 20-50% of patients after balloon angioplasty and in 10-30% of patients receiving a stent. Three distinct processes are involved—recoil of the vessel, neointimal proliferation, and early thrombus formation. The relative contribution of each of these depends on the type of injury. About three quarters of the lumen loss after balloon angioplasty is due to vessel recoil and the rest to neointimal proliferation,[2] whereas coronary stenting virtually eliminates vessel recoil, and restenosis is largely due to neointimal proliferation. Growth factors and cytokines are the major stimuli for proliferation of smooth muscle cells after an artery is injured, when deposition of platelets, leucocyte infiltration, expansion of smooth muscle cells, deposition of extracellular matrix, and re-endothelialisation occur. The platelets release platelet derived growth factor, transforming growth factor, epidermal growth factor, and thrombin, which stimulate the migration, growth, and division of smooth muscle cells.[w2 w3] Within the smooth muscle cell, cyclin dependent kinase and cyclins (regulators) drive the cell from one phase to another: G0, resting phase; G1, growth phase; S, replication of DNA; G2, preparation for division; and M, cell division. Cyclin dependent kinase has been described as the engine and the cyclins as the gearbox, determining whether the engine will run in the steady state or drive the cell forward in the cell cycle. Together they regulate cell

Box 1: Evolution of percutaneous interventions

- Phase 1 (1977-87): simple balloon angioplasty
- Phase 2 (1988-92): new device angioplasty
- Phase 3 (1993-2002): stent revolution

Restenosis and instent restenosis, 1977-2002

Year and procedure	Indications	Restenosis rate (%)	New problem	Solution
1977-87: percutaneous transluminal coronary angioplasty	Simple lesions, chronic syndromes	30-50	Restenosis, subacute closure	Stent
1988-92:				
Newer devices—Rotablater, excimer laser coronary angioplasty, directional coronary atherectomy	Complex, calcific, tortuous, bifurcations, left main, multiple lesions	50	Restenosis; restenosis 50-70%	Intravascular ultrasound guided use
Stents	Acute coronary syndromes	20-30	Restenosis, subacute thrombosis, instent restenosis	High pressure, anticoagulation
1993-2002: newer stents (biodegradable, covered, radioactive, intravascular ultrasonography)	Carotids, iliacs, renals, saphenous vein grafts, abdominal aortic aneurysms direct, rupture	10-20	Instent restenosis, re-restenosis 50-70%	Improved designs and material, radiation
1995-2002: brachytherapy—photodynamic therapy, ultrasonography, cryotherapy, cutting balloon	Instent restenosis	<10	Restenosis, re-restenosis10% late thrombosis, edge failure, geographical miss	Prolonged antiplatelets
2002: eluting stents—drugs, gene	Simple lesions, chronic syndromes, some complex lesions	0-5	?Delayed restenosis	?Ultimate angioplasty

cycle progression and migration of smooth muscle cells (figure).

Clinically significant restenosis generally occurs between one and three months after balloon angioplasty. Most patients present with typical angina, usually within four months of the procedure—restenosis is much less likely to be the cause of symptoms after six months. With coronary stenting the presentation is delayed further by about one to three months.[3 w4]

Prediction of restenosis

Restenosis depends on several factors (box 2). The risk of restenosis is increased in patients with diabetes mellitus, acute coronary syndromes, and, importantly, an inherent predisposition to restenosis.[4 w5 w6] The increased restenosis rate among patients with diabetes is attributed to endothelial dysfunction, dysregulation of growth factor production, and increased platelet aggregability and thrombogenicity.[w7] In acute coronary syndromes, vascular injury worsens the existing thrombogenic milieu and promotes cellular proliferation. Evidence of a predilection to restenosis comes from observations of a bimodal pattern of distribution of stenosis after angioplasty and the presence of restenosis at another treated site.[5 w8] This predisposition might be mediated by genetic factors. Putative abnormalities are deletion polymorphisms of the gene encoding angiotensin converting enzyme, abnormalities in the expression of genes encoding the platelet Gp IIb-IIIa receptors, and some specific apolipoprotein E genotypes.[w9 w10 w11] The most important lesion characteristics predicting restenosis are a small vessel diameter and a long lesion length.[6 7 w12 w13] A large minimum lumen diameter after stenting reduces the rate of restenosis—that is, "bigger is better."[w13]

Prevention of restenosis

Drugs

Several drugs, including those with antiplatelet, antithrombotic, antiproliferative, and anti-inflammatory properties, have been used to prevent restenosis, but except for probucol and prednisolone their contribution has been largely disappointing.[w14 w15] The role of drugs in preventing restenosis is likely to be small because the principal mechanism of restenosis after balloon angioplasty concerns remodelling of the artery. These drugs might have a role in preventing neointimal proliferation after stenting.

Coronary stents

Stents produce the largest net gain in lumen diameter because they achieve an immediate large gain with modest later loss of diameter. The Belgium Netherlands stent study (BENESTENT) and the stent restenosis study (STRESS) showed that stents reduce restenosis rates after balloon angioplasty.[8 9] These studies were conducted on "ideal" lesions, however, and higher restenosis rates have occurred with more complex lesions. Several materials, coatings, and designs have been developed in the quest for the ideal stent (see table A on bmj.com). Most have shown little success, except for drug eluting stents.

Drug eluting coronary stents

Using a coronary stent for local delivery of drugs combines scaffolding with targeted drug action. Although initial research and clinical trials concentrated on sirolimus and paclitaxel, numerous agents with antiproliferative properties are currently under investigation (see table B on bmj.com).

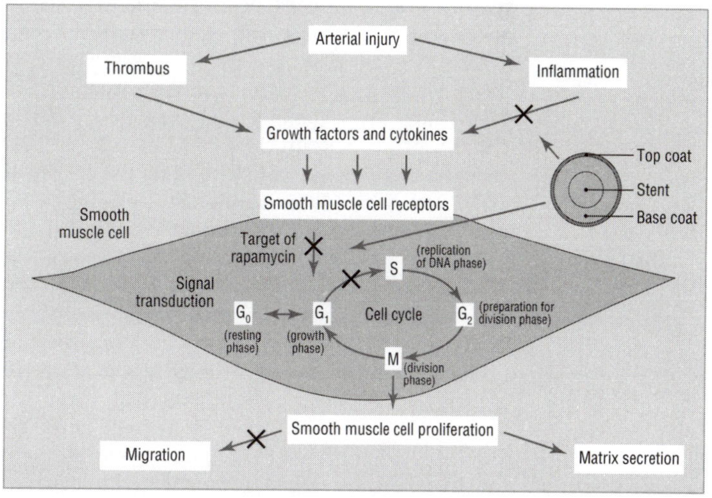

Inhibition of neointimal formation by sirolimus impregnated stent

Box 2: Predictors of restenosis

Patient factors

- Restenosis at another treated site
- Diabetes mellitus
- Intervention in acute coronary syndromes

Lesion characteristics and procedural variables

- Diameter of vessel
- Length of lesion or stent
- Minimum lumen diameter before stenting
- Minimum lumen diameter after stenting ("bigger is better")
- Ostial lesions
- Saphenous venous grafts
- Total occlusions

Sirolimus

Sirolimus (Rapamycin; Wyeth-Ayerst, PA, USA), a macrolide antibiotic with potent antifungal, immunosuppressive, and antimitotic properties, is produced by *Streptomyces hygroscopicus*, an actinomycete found in soil. It is used to prevent the rejection of renal transplants, but its systemic use is limited by the side effects of hyperlipidaemia and thrombocytopenia.[w16] Stents are coated with a polymer containing low dose sirolimus then a layer of drug-free polymer, which serves as a barrier to diffusion. The polymer acts as a reservoir for sirolimus, allowing gradual elution of the drug (see figure). Sirolimus downregulates cytokine dependent kinase mTOR (mammalian target of rapamycin), thus preventing progression from the G1 phase (cell growth) to the S phase (DNA replication).[10 11 w17] Sirolimus is only effective when bound to sirolimus binding protein (FKBP), present only on smooth muscle cells and lymphocytes, thereby providing important targeting.

In the initial pilot study of sirolimus (30 patients), the stent virtually eliminated angiographic and ultrasonic evidence of neointimal proliferation.[12 w18] No instent or edge restenosis (restenosis within the stent or within 5 mm proximal and distal to the stent edges) was noted, and no major complications occurred. In the randomised study with the sirolimus eluting Bx velocity balloon expandable stent in the treatment of patients with de novo native coronary artery lesions (RAVEL) study (238 patients), no restenosis was observed in the sirolimus stent group compared with 27% of patients in the uncoated stent group.[13] In the US arm of the SIRolImUS eluting stent in de novo native coronary lesions (SIRIUS) study, 9% of patients in the sirolumus stent group showed angiographic evidence of restenosis at nine months compared with 37% in the uncoated stent group.[w19] Revascularisation of the target lesion was reduced from 17% to 4%. There was no increase in subacute or late thrombosis. These results were all the more significant because many patients in this study were at a high risk of restenosis (patients with diabetes, those who had multivessel angioplasty, and those with overlapping stents). The Food and Drug Administration has recently approved the clinical use of sirolimus eluting stents in the United States.

Paclitaxel

Paclitaxel was originally isolated from the bark of the Pacific yew. It is an antineoplastic agent, currently used to treat ovarian cancer. Paclitaxel enhances the assembly of microtubules that interrupt proliferation, migration, and signal transduction. It is incorporated into a fast release carrier system on the stent. Trials of paclitaxel coated stents have shown significant reductions in restenosis. The pacliTAXel-elUting Stent (TAXUS I) trial showed no restenosis in the paclitaxel stent group at 12 months compared with 10% for the standard stent group.[14] This difference was reflected in the revascularisation of the target lesion in both groups (0% *v* 10%). The major adverse cardiac event rate at one year was also considerably reduced (3% *v* 10%). Results were maintained at 24 months. The TAXUS II trial confirmed the reduction in restenosis.[w20] Similar results were observed in the European evaluation of paclitaxel eluting stent trial (ELUTES).[w21] In the recently published Asian paclitaxel eluting stent clinical trial (ASPECT), angiographic restenosis decreased from 27% in the uncoated stent group to 4% in the paclitaxel stent group, due to a dose dependent decrease in neointimal proliferation.[w22] No increase in subacute stent thrombosis (thrombosis occurring between 48 hours and two weeks after stenting) or restenosis at the edges of the stent has been reported in published randomised trials. However, late thrombosis has been reported after stopping antiplatelet therapy.[w23] Some concern has been expressed that inflammation of the intima might occur at higher doses. Nevertheless, it is clear that drug eluting stents will be increasingly used for the prevention of restenosis because they nearly eliminate neointimal proliferation with little untoward effect and without the need for special expertise or instrumentation.

Biodegradable stents

The Japanese Igaki-Tamai stent is made of poly-L-lactic acid and takes 18-24 months to biodegrade. The scaffolding prevents abrupt vessel closure in the acute phase and vessel recoil within six months. Clinical results are available for 15 patients, showing no major complications and a restenosis rate of about 10%.[w24] The stent is being evaluated further.

Debulking devices

The occurrence of restenosis is reduced when larger minimum lumen diameters are achieved after stenting. This makes a case for the use of debulking devices to mechanically reduce plaque volume. Early trials comparing directional coronary atherectomy with balloon angioplasty showed an increased mortality and Q wave infarction with atherectomy.[15 w25] Subsequently, strategies to optimally debulk combined with adjunctive balloon angioplasty to achieve the largest possible lumen diameters were tested against conventional balloon angioplasty.[16w26] Less restenosis was shown with directional coronary atherectomy compared with plain balloon angioplasty, but there was no difference in revascularisation of the target vessel at one year. Further, this benefit came at the cost of a higher incidence of increases in periprocedural myocardial enzymes. This failure to show consistent benefit from debulking has been attributed to the late loss in lumen diameter being proportional to the acute gain after the procedure (device "taxing"). A synergistic approach using directional coronary atherectomy and coronary stenting might have a role in reducing restenosis rates in complex lesions.[w27 w28]

Gene therapy

Vascular gene therapy can potentially control cellular growth related restenosis by modifying gene expression. Antisense oligonucleotides can be used to block gene expression by binding segments of specific mRNA with complementary DNA sequences. In a porcine model of restenosis, intramural delivery of specific antisense oligonucleotides completely eliminated c-myc expression and dramatically reduced neointimal proliferation.[w29] An alternative approach is by transfer of genes, which have beneficial antiproliferative effects (for example, genes for endothelial nitric oxide synthase (eNOS) and vascular endothelial growth factor). Gene transfer has mostly been achieved using adenoviruses as vectors, although plasmid DNA and retroviruses have also been used. Animal studies with gene transfer have shown marked inhibition of neointimal proliferation; phase I studies in humans are under way.[w30]

Intracoronary radiation

The role of intracoronary radiation in preventing restenosis in de novo lesions is not entirely clear. Although one study showed a dose dependent decrease in the rate of restenosis after angioplasty, data from two studies in the United States were not favourable.[17 w31 w32]

Instent restenosis

Instent restenosis is due largely to neointimal proliferation. A classification for instent restenosis has been developed, depending on the degree and distribution of the hyperplastic neointima.[18] Broadly, instent restenosis can be focal or diffuse. Therapeutic success is dictated by the volume and extent of the neointima. Focal lesions respond much better than diffuse ones.

Balloon angioplasty

In contrast to the atherosclerotic plaque in de novo lesions, the hyperplastic neointima is relatively less compressible, and therefore the emphasis has been on debulking rather than on plaque compression to prevent recurrent stenosis. Nevertheless, balloon angioplasty has been used extensively. The occurrence of restenosis in this setting largely depends on whether the restenosis is focal or diffuse. The recurrent restenosis rate with diffuse lesions has been shown to be twice that of focal lesions (63% *v* 31%, respectively).[w33] However, the recent angioplasty versus rotational atherectomy for treatment of diffuse instent restenosis trial (ARTIST) suggests that even for diffuse lesions balloon angioplasty is better than rotational atherectomy.[19] Plain balloon angioplasty is also likely to be successful in patients with restenosis due to poorly apposed stent struts, where luminal gain depends more on additional stent expansion than tissue compression.[w34] A meta-analysis concluded that balloon angioplasty should be the procedure of choice when a good immediate outcome can be expected, because the nine month major adverse cardiac event rate is virtually identical with all forms of treatment.[w35] Additional stenting within the region of instent restenosis ("stent sandwich") improves immediate angiographic outcomes, but long term results are poor.[w36 w37]

Cutting balloon angioplasty

Cutting balloon angioplasty utilises a standard balloon catheter with three or four microblades (depth 0.18 mm, thickness 0.70-0.76 mm). The blades, attached longitudinally and folded within the balloon, are exposed on inflation and cut the neointimal tissue, facilitating plaque compression. They also help to anchor the balloon to the neointima (standard balloons tend to slip proximally or distally during inflation). Cutting balloon angioplasty for instent restenosis is associated with lower rates of revascularisation of target lesions and restenosis.[w38-w40] At many centres, cutting balloon angioplasty combined with intracoronary radiation is the treatment of choice for instent restenosis.

Debulking devices

Rotational atherectomy

Rotational atherectomy utilises a high speed (150 000-200 000 rpm) diamond tipped drill, which effectively removes hyperplastic neointima and results in a larger minimum lumen diameter compared with balloon angioplasty. The promising early results (20% restenosis) of the randomised trial of percutaneous transluminal coronary angioplasty versus rotablator for diffuse instent restenosis (ROSTER) could not be reproduced in the angioplasty versus rotational atherectomy for treatment of diffuse instent restenosis trial (ARTIST), which showed a worse outcome for rotablation.[19 w41] One possible reason for this discrepancy is that the low pressure used for inflation of the balloon after rotablation led to little increase in the stent diameter. Presumably high pressure inflation would resolve this.

Directional coronary atherectomy

Directional coronary atherectomy effectively removes neointima, with about a third of patients requiring revascularisation of target lesions at 10 months.[w42] However one meta-analysis showed that at nine months the major adverse cardiac event rates with directional coronary atherectomy did not differ significantly from other procedures.[w35] Further, activation of the cutter through stent struts may disrupt stent integrity or create sharp edges that puncture balloons.

Intracoronary radiation (brachytherapy)

A more recent approach to instent restenosis is intracoronary radiation or brachytherapy, on the grounds that it may control the excessive proliferative response and limit neointima formation, analogous to low doses of ionising radiation to treat benign proliferative disorders such as keloids, heterotropic bone formation, and pterygia.[w43] Different isotopes on various platforms have been used to develop practical systems for endovascular brachytherapy. The platforms are catheter based systems such as line source wires, radioactive beads (delivered hydraulically), and balloons filled with radioactive gas or liquid, or stents incorporating γ (low energy, high penetration) or β (high energy, low penetration) emitters.

The first intracoronary brachytherapy procedure in humans was performed in Caracas, Venezuela in 1994.[w44] Endovascular brachytherapy has since been tested in over 5000 patients, leading to approval by the Food and Drug Administration for the treatment of instent restenosis with both β and γ radiation.[w45]

Of the trials for the treatment of coronary instent restenosis by brachytherapy (see table C on bmj.com), the important ones are catheter based radiotherapy to inhibit restenosis after coronary stenting (SCRIPPS I), intracoronary gamma radiation therapy after angioplasty inhibits recurrence in patients with instent restenosis (WRIST), and localised intracoronary gamma radiation therapy to inhibit the recurrence of restenosis after stenting (GAMMA I).[20 21 w46] Initiated at the Scripps Clinic in March 1995, SCRIPPS I tested the efficacy of iridium-192 (γ source) in 55 patients with restenosis. At follow up, the patients who received radiation had better mean minimum lumen diameters, less late loss of lumen, and lower restenosis rates. The WRIST trial randomised 100 patients with instent restenosis and 30 patients with instent restenosis in saphenous vein grafts to ^{192}Ir or placebo. Restenosis was significantly reduced, particularly in patients with diabetes and those with vein grafts. Similarly, in the GAMMA I study on 252 patients, the primary end point—death, myocardial infarction, and the need for repeat revascularisation of the target lesion during nine months of follow up—occurred in 53 patients assigned to placebo (44%) and 37 patients assigned to ^{192}Ir (28%). Similar results have been observed with β radiation in the proliferation reduction with vascular energy trial (PREVENT) and intimal hyperplasia inhibition with beta in-stent trial (INHIBIT).[22 w47]

Two important complications related to brachytherapy are edge restenosis ("candy wrapper" effect) and the risk of late thrombosis. Edge restenosis was first noted with radioactive stents and is possibly the result of radiation dose "fall-off" at the edges of the stent combined with vessel wall injury from inflation of the balloon outside the stent margins. Edge restenosis may be prevented by avoiding the "geographic miss,"—that is, a portion of the vessel that has undergone injury during the procedure, but has not received the intended dose of radiation. The likelihood of geographic miss can be decreased by radioactive coverage of an adequate length of the vessel.[w48 w49]

Delayed (after one month) thrombosis may occur in up to 9% of patients receiving additional stents at the time of radiation.[23] Therefore, such repeat stenting (stent sandwich) is discouraged. Further, a long course (more than six months) of antiplatelet therapy is recommended for all patients undergoing brachytherapy. Such treatment has reduced the risk of late thrombosis to that of the control population.[w50]

Drug eluting coronary stents

Preliminary data on a paclitaxel coated stent has shown a high major adverse cardiac event rate, which was largely due to the need for repeat revascularisation of the target lesion.[w51] The potential for improved results with drug eluting stents in the treatment of instent restenosis is being explored.

Additional educational resources

Reviews

O'Neill WW, Leon MB. Drug-eluting stents: costs versus clinical benefit. *Circulation* 2003;107:3008-11.

Lemos PA, Serruys PW, Sousa JE. Drug-eluting stents: cost versus clinical benefit. *Circulation* 2003;107:3003-7.

Kandzari DE, Mark DB. Intracoronary brachytherapy: time to sell short? [Editorial.] *Circulation* 2002;106:646-8.

Website

tctmd (www.tctmd.com)—an industry supported website, providing useful information on topics in interventional cardiology.

Information for patients

Cypher, sirolimus eluting coronary stent (www.cypherusa.com/patient)—Patient section of Cordis Corporation's sirolimus eluting stent website. Provides useful general information about restenosis and drug eluting stents.

The future

Drug eluting coronary stents will be increasingly used in clinical practice despite their high initial cost (about three times that of a bare metal stent) because the cost is likely to be compensated for by the reduced need for repeat revascularisation. The costs of stents should go down as more manufacturers enter the market, especially from Asia. It is anticipated that under 5% of patients who undergo multivessel angioplasty will need repeat revascularisation compared with the current 14-16%. This is expected to at least equal, if not better, the outcome with coronary artery bypass surgery for patients with multivessel disease, even in those with diabetes. This will be tested in the arterial revascularisation therapies (ARTS II) study.[24] Intracoronary brachytherapy will remain the best treatment for diffuse or refractory instent restenosis[w52] until drug eluting stents are proved useful for this indication or until an efficient and reliable antiproliferative genetic therapy becomes available.

Contributors: All authors were involved in the preparation of the manuscript and in the revision process. BB will act as guarantor.

Funding: None declared.

Competing interests: None declared.

1 Gruntzig A. Transluminal dilation of coronary artery stenosis. *Lancet* 1978;1:263.
2 Mintz GS, Popma JJ, Pichard AD, Kent KM, Satler LF, Wong C, et al. Arterial remodeling after coronary angioplasty: a serial intravascular ultrasound study. *Circulation* 1996;94:35-43.
3 Serruys PW, Luijten HE, Beatt KJ, Geuskens R, de Feyter PJ, van den Brand M, et al. Incidence of restenosis after successful coronary angioplasty: a time-related phenomenon. A quantitative angiographic study in 342 consecutive patients at 1, 2, 3, and 4 months. *Circulation* 1988;77:361-71.
4 Abizaid A, Kornowski R, Mintz GS, Hong MK, Abizaid AS, Mehran R, et al. The influence of diabetes mellitus on acute and late clinical outcomes following coronary stent implantation. *J Am Coll Cardiol* 1998;32:584-9.
5 Schomig A, Kastrati A, Elezi S, Schuhlen H, Dirschinger J, Dannegger F, et al. Bimodal distribution of angiographic measures of restenosis six months after coronary stent placement. *Circulation* 1997;96:3880-7.
6 Hirshfeld JW Jr, Schwartz JS, Jugo R, MacDonald RG, Goldberg S, Savage MP, et al. Restenosis after coronary angioplasty: a multivariate statistical model to relate lesion and procedure variables to restenosis. The M-HEART Investigators. *J Am Coll Cardiol* 1991;18:647-56.
7 Kuntz RE, Gibson CM, Nobuyoshi M, Baim DS. Generalized model of restenosis after conventional balloon angioplasty, stenting and directional atherectomy. *J Am Coll Cardiol* 1993;21:15-25.
8 Serruys PW, de Jaegere P, Kiemeneij F, Macaya C, Rutsch W, Heyndrickx G, et al. A comparison of balloon-expandable stent implantation with balloon angioplasty in patients with coronary artery disease. *N Engl J Med* 1994;331:489-95.

9 Fischman DL, Leon MB, Baim DS, Schatz RA, Savage MP, Penn I, et al. A randomized comparison of coronary-stent placement and balloon angioplasty in the treatment of coronary artery disease. *N Engl J Med* 1994;331:496-501.

10 Marx SO, Jayaraman T, Go LO, Marks AR. Rapamycin-FKBP inhibits cell cycle regulators of proliferation in vascular smooth muscle cells. *Circ Res* 1995;76:412-7.

11 Poon M, Marx SO, Gallo R, Badimon JJ, Taubman MB, Marks AR. Rapamycin inhibits vascular smooth muscle cell migration. *J Clin Invest* 1996;98:2277-83.

12 Sousa JE, Costa MA, Abizaid A, Abizaid AS, Feres F, Pinto IM, et al. Lack of neointima proliferation after implantation of sirolimus-coated stents in human coronary arteries: a quantitative coronary angiography and three dimensional intravascular ultrasound study. *Circulation* 2001;103:192-5.

13 Morice MC, Serruys PW, Sousa JE, Fajadet J, Ban Hayashi E, Perin M, et al. Randomized study with the sirolimus-coated Bx velocity balloon-expandable stent in the treatment of patients with de novo native coronary artery lesions. A randomized comparison of a sirolimus-eluting stent with a standard stent for coronary revascularization. *N Engl J Med* 2002;346:1773-80.

14 Grube E, Silber S, Hauptmann KE, Mueller R, Buellesfeld L, Gerckens U, et al. TAXUS I: six- and twelve-month results from a randomized, double-blind trial on a slow-release paclitaxel-eluting stent for de novo coronary lesions. *Circulation* 2003;107:38-42.

15 Elliot JM, Berdan LG, Holmes DR, Isner JM, King SB, Keeler GP, et al. One-year follow-up in the coronary angioplasty versus excisional atherectomy trial (CAVEAT I). *Circulation* 1995;91:2158-66.

16 Simonton CA, Leon MB, Baim DS, Hinohara T, Kent KM, Bersin RM, et al. 'Optimal' directional coronary atherectomy: final results of the optimal atherectomy restenosis study (OARS). *Circulation* 1998;97:332-9.

17 Verin V, Popowski Y, de Bruyne B, Baumgart D, Sauerwein W, Lins M, et al. Endoluminal beta-radiation therapy for the prevention of coronary restenosis after balloon angioplasty. The Dose-Finding Study Group. *N Engl J Med* 2001;344:243-9.

18 Mehran R, Dangas G, Abizaid AS, Mintz GS, Lansky AJ, Satler LF, et al. Angiographic patterns of in-stent restenosis: classification and implications for long term outcome. *Circulation* 1999;100:1872-8.

19 vom Dahl J, Dietz U, Haager PK, Silber S, Niccoli L, Buettner HJ, et al. Rotational atherectomy does not reduce recurrent in-stent restenosis: results of the angioplasty versus rotational atherectomy for treatment of diffuse in-stent restenosis trial (ARTIST). *Circulation* 2002;105:583-8.

20 Teirstein PS, Massullo V, Jani S, Popma JJ, Mintz GS, Russo RJ, et al. Catheter-based radiotherapy to inhibit restenosis after coronary stenting (SCRIPPS). *N Engl J Med* 1997;336:1697-703.

21 Leon MB, Teirstein PS, Moses JW, Tripuraneni P, Lansky AJ, Jani S, et al. Localized intracoronary gamma-radiation therapy to inhibit the recurrence of restenosis after stenting (GAMMA I). *N Engl J Med* 2001;344:250-6.

22 Waksman R, Raizner AE, Yeung AC, Lansky AJ, Vandertie L on behalf of the INHIBIT Investigators. Use of localized intracoronary β radiation in the treatment of instent restenosis: the INHIBIT randomized controlled trial. *Lancet* 2002;359:551-7.

23 Waksman R, Bhargava B, Mintz GS, Mehran R, Lansky AJ, Leon MB. Late total occlusion following intracoronary brachytherapy for patients with instent restenosis. *J Am Coll Cardiol* 2000;36:65-8.

24 Serruys PW. ARTS I—the rapamycin eluting stent; ARTS II—the rosy prophecy. *Eur Heart J* 2002;23:757-9.

(Accepted 3 July 2003)

ISBN 0-929661-90-7
ISSN 1542-1368
Twelfth Printing
Printed in the United States of America

The Johns Hopkins White Papers are published yearly by Medletter Associates, Inc.

The 2004 White Papers

Take Control of Your Medical Condition

Visit us online at www.HopkinsAfter50.com

64B60M

YES, I've placed a check mark next to the White Paper(s) I'd like to receive for $24.95 each. Annual updates on each subject that I have chosen will be offered to me by announcement card. I need do nothing if I want the update to be sent to me automatically. If I do not want it, I will return the announcement card marked "cancel." I may cancel at any time. (Please add $2.95 for domestic, $4.95 for Canadian, and $15.00 for foreign orders to your total to cover shipping and handling.) (Florida residents add sales tax.)

✔ **Please put a check mark next to the White Paper(s) you wish to order.**

Code		Title	Price
001040	❑	Arthritis	$24.95
003046	❑	Coronary Heart Disease	$24.95
004044	❑	Depression and Anxiety	$24.95
005041	❑	Diabetes	$24.95
006049	❑	Hypertension and Stroke	$24.95
007047	❑	Nutrition and Weight Control for Longevity	$24.95
008045	❑	Prostate Disorders	$24.95
010041	❑	Digestive Disorders	$24.95
011049	❑	Vision	$24.95
012047	❑	Back Pain & Osteoporosis	$24.95
015040	❑	Memory	$24.95
019042	❑	Lung Disorders	$24.95
020040	❑	Heart Attack Prevention	$24.95

METHOD OF PAYMENT: (U.S. funds only) ❑ VISA ❑ Check Enclosed ❑ MasterCard ❑ Bill Me

Name

Address

City State Zip

Credit Card # Exp. Date

Signature Date

Money Back Guarantee: If for any reason, you are not satisfied after receipt of your publications, return your purchase within 30 days for a full refund.

Detach and mail this card back to The Johns Hopkins White Papers, P.O. Box 420083, Palm Coast, FL 32142

The 2004 White Papers

Take Control of Your Medical Condition

Visit us online at www.HopkinsAfter50.com

64B60M

YES, I've placed a check mark next to the White Paper(s) I'd like to receive for $24.95 each. Annual updates on each subject that I have chosen will be offered to me by announcement card. I need do nothing if I want the update to be sent to me automatically. If I do not want it, I will return the announcement card marked "cancel." I may cancel at any time. (Please add $2.95 for domestic, $4.95 for Canadian, and $15.00 for foreign orders to your total to cover shipping and handling.) (Florida residents add sales tax.)

✔ **Please put a check mark next to the White Paper(s) you wish to order.**

Code		Title	Price
001040	❑	Arthritis	$24.95
003046	❑	Coronary Heart Disease	$24.95
004044	❑	Depression and Anxiety	$24.95
005041	❑	Diabetes	$24.95
006049	❑	Hypertension and Stroke	$24.95
007047	❑	Nutrition and Weight Control for Longevity	$24.95
008045	❑	Prostate Disorders	$24.95
010041	❑	Digestive Disorders	$24.95
011049	❑	Vision	$24.95
012047	❑	Back Pain & Osteoporosis	$24.95
015040	❑	Memory	$24.95
019042	❑	Lung Disorders	$24.95
020040	❑	Heart Attack Prevention	$24.95

METHOD OF PAYMENT: (U.S. funds only) ❑ VISA ❑ Check Enclosed ❑ MasterCard ❑ Bill Me

Name

Address

City State Zip

Credit Card # Exp. Date

Signature Date

Money Back Guarantee: If for any reason, you are not satisfied after receipt of your publications, return your purchase within 30 days for a full refund.

Detach and mail this card back to The Johns Hopkins White Papers, P.O. Box 420083, Palm Coast, FL 32142

Johns Hopkins White Papers

Fold along this line and tape closed

NO POSTAGE NECESSARY IF MAILED IN THE UNITED STATES

BUSINESS REPLY MAIL
FIRST-CLASS MAIL PERMIT NO. 86 FLAGLER BEACH FL

POSTAGE WILL BE PAID BY ADDRESSEE

THE JOHNS HOPKINS WHITE PAPERS
PO BOX 420083
PALM COAST FL 32142-9264

Johns Hopkins White Papers

Fold along this line and tape closed

NO POSTAGE NECESSARY IF MAILED IN THE UNITED STATES

BUSINESS REPLY MAIL
FIRST-CLASS MAIL PERMIT NO. 86 FLAGLER BEACH FL

POSTAGE WILL BE PAID BY ADDRESSEE

THE JOHNS HOPKINS WHITE PAPERS
PO BOX 420083
PALM COAST FL 32142-9264

2004 WHITE PAPER TITLES

ARTHRITIS 2004 - Covers three common forms of arthritis - osteoarthritis, rheumatoid arthritis, and gout - as well as two other rheumatic diseases: fibromyalgia syndrome and bursitis.

CORONARY HEART DISEASE 2004 - Discusses four problems resulting from coronary heart disease: heart attacks, angina, cardiac arrhythmias, and heart failure.

DEPRESSION and ANXIETY 2004 - Includes major depression, dysthymia, atypical depression, bipolar disorder, seasonal affective disorder, panic disorder, generalized anxiety disorder, obsessive-compulsive disorder, post-traumatic stress disorder, and phobic disorders.

DIABETES 2004 - Shows you how to manage your diabetes and avoid complications such as foot problems and vision changes. Reviews the latest tools for monitoring your blood glucose and the newest medications for controlling it.

DIGESTIVE DISORDERS 2004 - Covers gastroesophageal reflux disease, peptic ulcers, dysphagia, achalasia, Barrett's esophagus, esophageal spasm and stricture, gastritis, gallstones, diarrhea, constipation, Crohn's disease, ulcerative colitis, and colon cancer.

HYPERTENSION and STROKE 2004 - Explains how to treat your high blood pressure and prevent it from harming your health. Also covers the two forms of stroke: ischemic stroke and hemorrhagic stroke.

BACK PAIN and OSTEOPOROSIS 2004 - Addresses back pain due to sprains, strains, and spasms; degenerative changes of the spinal bones and disks; disk herniation; and spinal stenosis. Also covers osteoporosis, a common cause of fractures in the spine and hip.

LUNG DISORDERS 2004 - Includes information on emphysema and chronic bronchitis (together referred to as chronic obstructive pulmonary disease or COPD), asthma, pneumonia, tuberculosis, lung cancer, and sleep apnea.

MEMORY 2004 - Tells you how to keep your memory sharp as you get older, and how to recognize the symptoms of age-associated memory impairment, mild cognitive impairment, and illnesses such as Alzheimer's disease and vascular dementia.

NUTRITION and WEIGHT CONTROL for LONGEVITY 2004 - Gives you the information you need to eat a healthy diet and keep your weight under control. Also explains what to do when the pounds just don't seem to budge.

PROSTATE DISORDERS 2004 - Helps you decide among the various treatment options for prostate cancer, benign prostatic hyperplasia, and prostatitis.

VISION 2004 - Reviews the current knowledge on cataracts, glaucoma, age-related macular degeneration, and diabetic retinopathy. Also discusses ways to cope with low vision.

HEART ATTACK PREVENTION 2004 - Provides up-to-date strategies for preventing a first heart attack, including identifying possible risk factors, the latest screening tests, risk-reducing lifestyle measures, and medications for controlling cholesterol.